Instant Pot Cookbook
for Beginners

Easy, Healthy and Fast Instant Pot Recipes
Anyone Can Cook

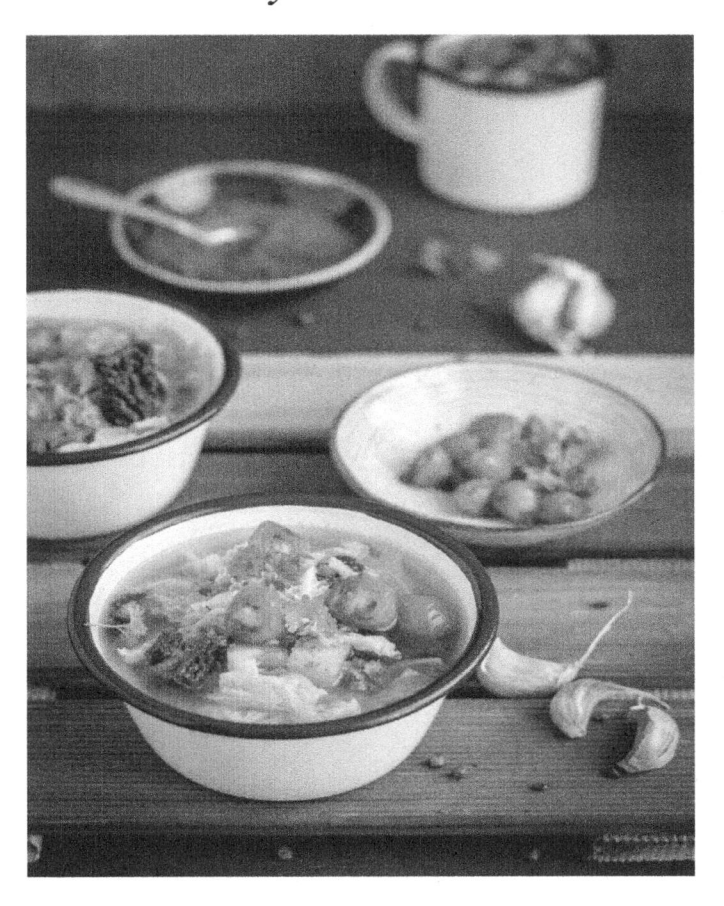

Alice Newman

Copyright © 2018 Alice Newman

All rights reserved

ISBN-13: 978-1985882072

ISBN-10: 1985882078

Dedication

For you, for your family, for everyone who wants to make sure they have easy and delicious meals to maintain a healthy lifestyle

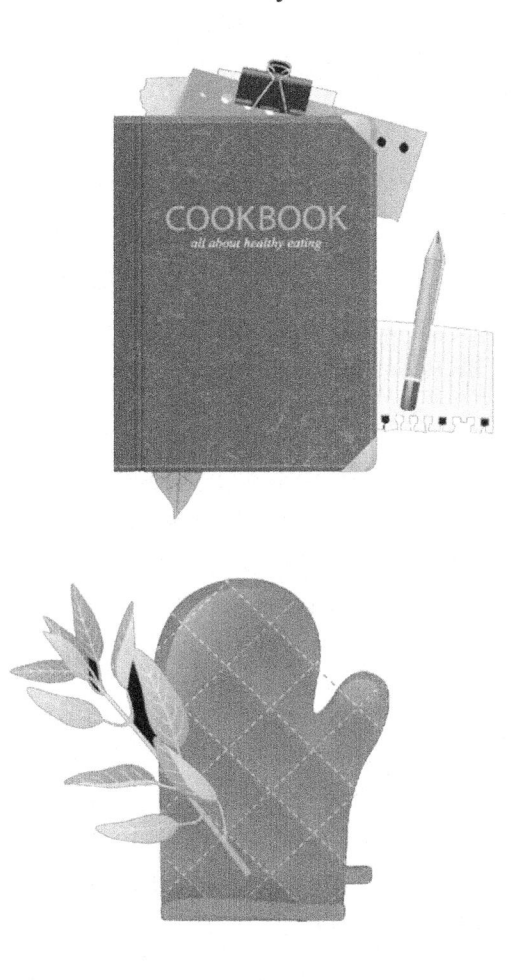

WHAT IS AN INSTANT POT

This amazing device can cook any meal—and it could be freaking fast. Instant Pot is simple enough for a 3-year-old to use, and you can be sure it can be the best help to you in your kitchen. In addition to cooking meals such as meat, chicken, beef, and dried beans at lightning speed, it also moonlights as a yogurt maker and a rice cooker. We could easily call it the Only Pot instead of the Instant Pot, since it's the only cooking device you need.

All of which means one very important thing: Cooking healthy, easy, mouthwatering meals has never been easier.

Once you have a full understanding of what the electric pressure cooker is and what it can do, you are going to fall in love with your newfound freedom in the kitchen. I am not joking, it's true.

The Instant Pot is a combination of seven different kitchen gadgets, and it can do far more than any one of those gadgets ever does on their own. Of course, this pressure cooker is very intimidating and can be downright confusing first, but with a little instruction, you will know what you're doing.

Your Instant Pot comes with an owner's manual, which is going to explain all the different buttons you see on the front of your gadget. Many of these buttons are already labeled, telling you up front what they do, and what you can do, but it's always nice to know the full capabilities, and limitations, of your new gadget before you get started.

You can make virtually anything you can think of with this pressure cooking device. With a variety of different settings built in, along with two separate levels of pressure cooking, you really can choose how you want things done.

This book holds more than 100 different recipes for you and your family to try.

Once you break through the basics and get used to how your new kitchen gadget works, you will open the floodgates to all the things you can do.

Of course, this book focuses on meat recipes, as you can see the Instant Pot has settings specifically for meat, but you can use this tool to your vegan foods and I have also included some vegetarian recipes.

The number one thing you will fall in love with is the versatility, and that is the most important aspect I wanted to celebrate in this book.

Regardless of how you choose to eat, you are going to find that this kitchen gadget has so many more features to it than you ever thought a single device could have, and as such, you have options.

The last thing you should know about the Instant Pot is that it is very safe in use, so you don't have to worry about anything. It's also *intelligent, convenient and dependable*.

With the Instant Pot, you can be sure that you can have the freedom to get your food cooking, and then go about your day. The entire gadget is designed to run off a timer, and the pot will change its pressure and heat based on the setting you have chosen.

Though the food and the container itself can get scorching hot, it's always nice to know that you can enjoy cooking with the item rather than having to stress about watching it the entire time you are cooking in the kitchen.

The Instant Pot has been designed for the busy mom or dad and will do wonders for your insane schedule.

Take fixing and forgetting to the next level with your Electric Pressure Cooker, and enjoy cooking as you used to.

Now, let's dive into the wonderful world of benefits, delicious meals, and how you can personally use the Instant Pot in a way that helps you.

However, be warned, you will be absolutely amazed. =)

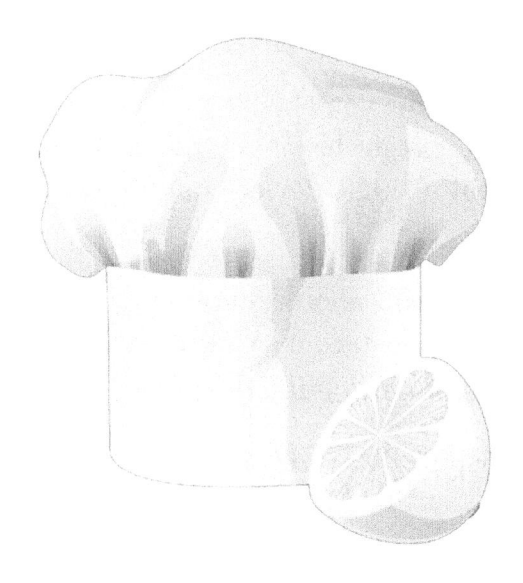

Table of Contents

Chicken Recipes 1

    Easy Faux Rotisserie Chicken 2

    Quick Adobo Chicken 3

    New Sesame Chicken 4

    Chili Lime Chicken Thighs 5

    Healthy Chicken Roast 6

    Chicken Curry with Mango 7

    Amazing Orange Chicken 8

    Salsa Chicken 9

    Healthy Buffalo Chicken 10

    Super Easy Citrus Herb Chicken 11

    Homemade Italian Shredded Chicken 12

    Mouthwatering Chicken Breasts with Lemon 13

    Mojo Chicken 14

    Spicy Chicken Curry with Coconut 15

    Quick All-in-one with Chicken and Rice 16

Beef Recipes 17

    Mouthwatering Garlic Meatballs 18

    Homemade Spaghetti Squash and Meat Sauce 19

    Healthy Corned Beef 20

    Easy Korean Beef 21

    Delicious Braised Short Ribs 22

Healthy Beef with Broccoli 23

Delicious Beef Stroganoff 25

Easy Mongolian Beef 26

Delicious Beef Stew 27

Beef Bourguignon 28

Red Wine Braised Beef Stew 29

Special Beef with Vegetables and Rice 30

Healthy Pot Roast 31

French Dip Sandwiches 32

Cheeseburger Macaroni 34

Pork, Turkey and Lamb Recipes 35

Instant Pulled Pork 36

Dr. Pepper Pulled Pork 37

Easy Instant BBQ Ribs 38

Delicious Rich Creamy Pork Chops 39

Tex-Mex Chili Mac 40

Simple Pork Adobo 41

Amazing Pork Carnitas 42

Quick and Easy Pork Chops 43

Instant Turkey Breast 44

Mouthwatering DIY Sandwiches 45

Homemade Cabbage Turkey Sausage 46

Healthy Turkey Verde & Rice 47

Delicious Lamb Stew 48

Super Easy Lamb Curry 49

Lamb Rogan Josh 50

Vegetable Recipes 51

Veggie Cauli Rice 52

Delicious Lentils in the Instant Pot 53

Curried Peas Curry 54

Simple Pinto Beans 55

Healthy Brussels Sprouts 56

Super Simple & Sweet Brussels Sprouts 57

Easy Baked Potato 58

Delicious Mashed Potatoes with Rosemary 59

Quick Mango Mashed Potatoes 60

Mushrooms with Green Beans and Bacon 61

Quick Asparagus Dinner 62

Delicious Mashed Sweet Potato 63

Simple Corn on the Cob 64

Delicious Pinto Bean Mash 65

Mouthwatering Smothered Cajun Greens 66

Rice and Quinoa Recipes 67

Chipotle's Cilantro Lime Rice 68

Delicious Coconut Lime Quinoa 69

Quick and Easy Quinoa 70

Delicious Parmesan Risotto 71

Easy Spanish Rice 72

Dessert Recipes **73**

Delicious Vanilla Bean Cheesecake 74

Simple Brownie Cake 75

Paleo Chocolate Cake 76

Healthy Apple Crisp 77

Mouthwatering Orange Cheesecake 78

Pina Colada Rice Pudding 80

Delicious Pumpkin Pies 81

Easy Oreo Cheesecake 82

Delicious Tapioca Pudding 84

Easy Banana Bread 85

Soup Recipes **86**

Butternut Squash Soup 87

Curried Butternut Squash Soup 88

Healthy Keto Chili 89

Bean and Sausage Soup 90

Taco Beef Soup 91

Homemade Seafood Gumbo 92

Quick Broccoli Soup 93

Easy Chicken Soup 94

Healthy Carrot Soup 95

Tomato Soup 96

Kale Soup with Chicken and Sweet Potato 97

Homemade Beef Paleo Stew 98

Apple Soup with Butternut Squash 99

Broccoli and Cheddar Soup 100

Easy Chicken Noodle Soup with Spinach 101

Easy Beef and Leek Soup 102

Breakfast Recipes 103

Healthy Coconut Yogurt 104

Oatmeal with Caramelized Bananas 105

Easy Homemade Oats 106

Healthy Instant Oats with Fruit 107

Energetic Boiled Egg 108

Banana French Toast 109

Delicious Scotch Eggs 110

Delicious Yogurt with Fruit 111

Breakfast Quinoa 112

Easy Buckwheat Porridge 113

CONCLUSION 114

Chicken Recipes

Easy Faux Rotisserie Chicken

Overall cooking time: 40 min

Servings: 4

Nutrition info: Calories: 396, fat: 28g, Carbs: 9g, protein: 26g.

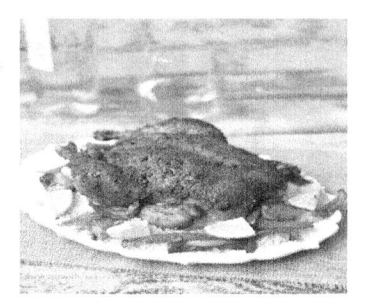

Ingredients:

Whole chicken	3 lbs.
Olive oil	2 tbsp.
Salt and pepper	to taste
Onion	½ medium
Garlic	5 cloves
Seasoning mix	3 tbsp.
Chicken stock	1 cup

Cooking procedure:

1. Take the chicken first, rub with olive oil, and sprinkle a pinch of pepper and salt. Place the garlic cloves and the onion inside the chicken and secure the legs with butcher's twine.
2. Now switch the pressure cooker on to sauté and add the remaining olive oil to the metal pan. Add the chicken and sauté both sides. Set aside.
3. Place the trivet and add the chicken stock. Sprinkle the seasoning mix over the chicken, rub and place the chicken in the cooker.
4. Close the lid and cook for 25 minutes. Remove the chicken from the cooker and allow cooling before Servings.

Quick Adobo Chicken

Overall cooking time: 30 min

Servings: 6

Nutrition info: Calories: 520, fat: 27g, Carbs: 29g, protein: 25g.

Ingredients:

Boneless chicken	2 lbs.
Seasoning	1 tbsp.
Turmeric	1 tbsp.
Tomatoes	4, chopped
Green chilies	7oz.
Water	½ cup

Cooking procedure:

1. First, place the chicken into the instant pot cooker and then sprinkle the seasoning over both sides of the chicken and rub evenly.
2. Now add the tomatoes and the chilies and then pour the water over the chicken.
3. Set the cooking time to 25 minutes, and cook with the lid on securely.
4. Shred the chicken with the help of two forks and stir with the juices in the pan to coat.
5. Serve with rice.

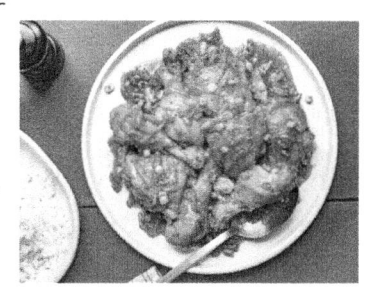

New Sesame Chicken

Overall cooking time: 10 min

Servings: 6

Nutrition info: Calories: 260, fat: 2g, Carbs: 10g, protein: 36g sodium: 0.8g.

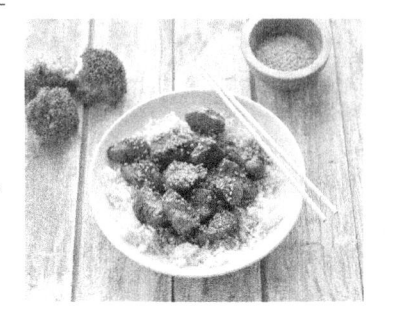

Ingredients:

Skinless chicken breasts	1.5 lbs.
Honey	¼ cup
Tamari	¼ cup
Minced garlic	1 tbsp.
Cornstarch	2 tbsp.
Red pepper	1 tsp.
Sesame seeds	1 tbsp.

Cooking procedure:

1. Switch the cooker to sauté and spread 1 tbsp. Olive oil over the pan of the cooker. Place the half of the chicken and sauté both sides. Do the same for the second half.
2. Take a mixing bowl and mix the all sauce ingredients together.
3. Place the chicken in the cooker and pour the sauce over it. Gently cover the chicken with sauce. Close the lid and set the slow cooker to chicken and cook for 4 minutes.
4. Remove the chicken after releasing the pressure and serve when it is hot with rice.

Chili Lime Chicken Thighs

Overall cooking time: 45 min

Servings: 5

Nutrition info: Calories: 120, fat: 3g, Carbs: 7g, protein: 15g, sodium: 105mg.

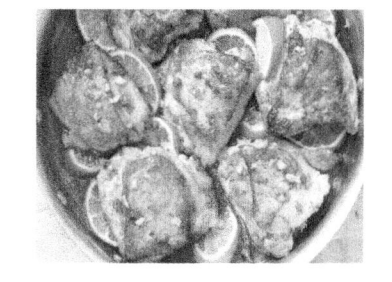

Ingredients:

Chicken thighs	4.
Olive oil	2 tbsp.
Garlic cloves	3
Cumin	1 tsp.
Chili powder	1 tbsp.
Cilantro	¼ cup, chopped
Chicken stock	½ cup
Arrowroot powder	1 tbsp.

Cooking procedure:

1. Take a mixing bowl and place the chili powder, cumin, garlic, lime juice and olive oil. Mix. Place the chicken into the mixture and pat well. Leave for 30 minutes.
2. Switch your pressure cooker to sauté and place 1 tbsp olive oil in the pan, then add the chicken thighs. Sauté both sides evenly.
3. Now add the chicken stock to the cooker, press the poultry switch, and set the time to 12 minutes.
4. Meanwhile, in a mixing cup, add the arrowroot powder with 2 tbsp. of water and mix well.
5. When the chicken is done, add the arrowroot mixture and cook for 8-10 minutes to thick the sauce mixture.
6. Serve with sauce immediately.

Healthy Chicken Roast

Overall cooking time: 45 min

Servings: 4

Nutrition info: Calories: 250, fat: 31g, Carbs: 1g, protein: 30g, sodium: 0.7g.

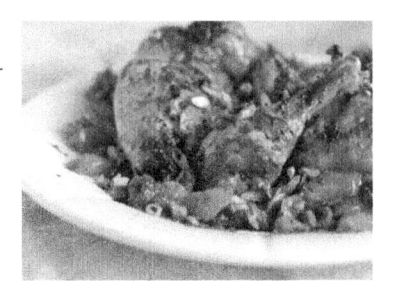

Ingredients:

Whole chicken	1.
Olive oil	1 tbsp.
Lemon juice	1 tbsp.
Rosemary	2 tbsp.
Thyme	1 tbsp.
Sea salt	1 tbsp.
Black pepper	½ tbsp.
Bay leaf	1

Cooking procedure:

1. Switch on the pressure cooker to sauté and add the olive oil to the metal pan. Add the chicken and sauté both sides. Set aside.
2. Place the trivet and add the chicken stock, lemon juice, rosemary, and thyme. Sprinkle the salt and pepper over the chicken.
3. Close the lid, press the button for poultry and cook for 25 to 30 minutes. Remove the chicken from the cooker and allow cooling before serving with bay leaf.

Chicken Curry with Mango

Overall cooking time: 30 min

Servings: 6

Nutrition info: Calories: 320, fat: 15g, Carbs: 17g, protein: 31g, sodium: 224mg.

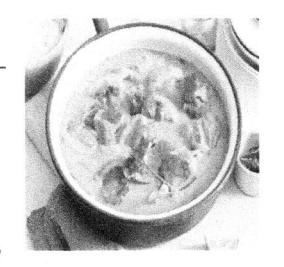

Ingredients:

Ghee	2 tbsp.	Chicken thighs	3 lbs.
Onion	1, sliced	Cauliflower	½ head
Garlic	3 tbsp.	Sweet potatoes	2
Tomato paste	3 tbsp.	Chicken stock	1 cup
Kosher salt	2 tbsp.	Coconut oil	1400ml
Curry powder	2 tbsp.	Baby spinach	3 cups
Cumin	2 tbsp.	Lime juice	1/2
Turmeric	1 tbsp.	Cilantro	½ cup
Cayenne	1/2 tbsp.	Mango	
Paprika	1/2 tbsp.		

Cooking procedure:

1. Switch the pressure cooker on to sauté and add the ghee, curry powder, salt, tomato paste, garlic, onion, cayenne, and paprika. Sauté for 4 minutes.
2. Now add the chicken thighs and stir. Add the sweet potatoes and cauliflower too. Stir well.
3. Add the chicken stock, close the lid, and set the cooking time to 20 minutes.
4. After cooking, add the frozen mango, lime juice, and baby spinach and stir evenly.

Amazing Orange Chicken

Overall cooking time: 30 min

Servings: 8

Nutrition info: Calories: 165, fat: 8g, Carbs: 14g, protein: 10g, sodium: 348mg.

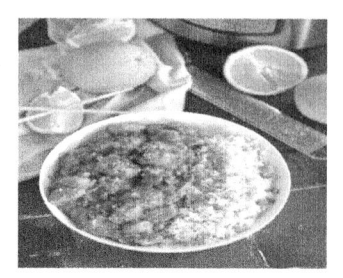

Ingredients:

Chicken breasts	4, boneless
Orange juice	1 cup
Orange zest	1 tbsp.
Garlic	3 tbsp.
Tamari	3 tbsp.
Honey	3 tbsp.
Rice vinegar	3 tbsp.
Sesame oil	1 tbsp.
Sriracha sauce	1 tbsp.
Brown sugar	¼ cup
Cornstarch	2 tbsp.

Cooking procedure:

1. Set the instant pot to sauté temperature and add chicken with sesame oil, sauté for 3 minutes. Add the garlic, ginger and the orange in the cooker, close the lid, and set the cooking time to 5 minutes on high.
2. Meanwhile, heat the rice with water on a stove.
3. While, the chicken is cooking, release the pressure, open the lid, add the cornstarch to the cooker and cook to thicken the sauce.
4. Serve with cooked rice.

Salsa Chicken

Overall cooking time: 15 min

Servings: 6

Nutrition info: Calories: 150, fat: 2g, Carbs: 5g, protein: 26g, sodium: 0.45g.

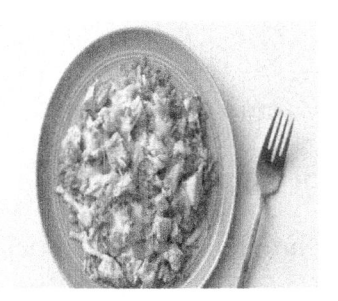

Ingredients:

Chicken breasts	2 lbs.
Goya salsa verde	17.6oz.
Chili	1 ½ tsp.
Cumin	1 ½ tbsp.
Paprika	1 tbsp.
Salt	1 tbsp.
Pepper	1 tbsp.
Jalapeno	1, diced
Onion	½, diced
Fresh cilantro	¼ cup, chopped
Lime	1

Cooking procedure:

1. Place half salsa verde in the instant pot and add the salt and pepper. Add the onion, cilantro, and the jalapeno and then add the chicken breasts.
2. ¼ cup of salsa set aside and pour remaining on the chicken. Close the lid and set the time for 10 minutes over high heat.
3. When the cooking is done, shred the chicken breasts using two forks and place in the pot for absorbing liquids.
4. Now pour the remaining salsa verde and lime. Mix evenly.

Healthy Buffalo Chicken

Overall cooking time: 20 min

Servings: 3-4

Nutrition info: Calories: 140, fat: 0.1g, Carbs: 5.1g, protein: 25g, sodium: 0.85g.

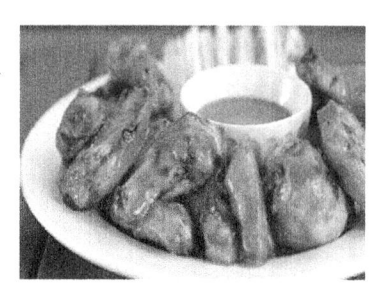

Ingredients:

Chicken breasts	4
Unsalted butter	4 tbsp.
Buffalo wing sauce	½ bottle
Honey	2 tbsp.
Tabasco sauce	2 tbsp.

Cooking procedure:

1. Place all the ingredients in your instant pot.
2. Switch on the pressure cooker to the manual setting for 10 minutes on high pressure and cook.
3. Shred the breasts by using two forks and allow absorption of the liquid in the instant pot.
4. Now switch the instant pot to sauté setting and sauté for another 5 minutes.

Super Easy Citrus Herb Chicken

Overall cooking time: 45 min

Servings: 4

Nutrition info: Calories: 250, fat: 31g, Carbs: 1g, protein: 30g, sodium: 0.7g.

Ingredients:

Grass-fed butter	3 tbsp.
Bone in chicken thighs	4
Salt	1 ½ tbsp.
Yellow onion	1 medium, sliced
Garlic	4 cloves
Thyme springs	5
Chorizo	½ lb.
Tomatoes	1/3 cup
Pitted green olives	½ cup
Orange juice	1/3 cup
Chicken bone broth	¾ cup
Cilantro	handful

Cooking procedure:

1. Switch the pressure cooker to sauté and pour two tablespoons of olive oil into the cooker. Insert the chicken thighs and sauté for 5 minutes on both sides with salt and pepper. Set aside.
2. Place the thyme leaves, onion, and the garlic with a little of the fat of your choice and sauté for another 5 minutes. Add the chorizo at the latter half of the sauté time.
3. Now add the chicken, olives, tomatoes, bone broth and orange juice and set the time for 20 minutes.
4. Serve immediately.

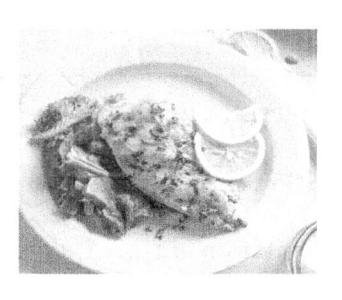

Homemade Italian Shredded Chicken

Overall cooking time: 15 min

Servings: 8

Nutrition info: Calories: 170, fat: 7g, Carbs: 0.03g, protein: 27g, sodium: 0g.

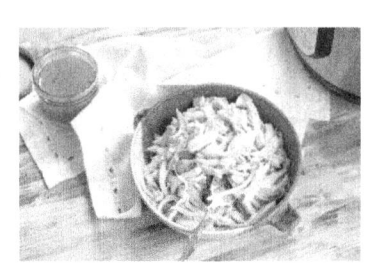

Ingredients:

Chicken breasts	4 lbs.
Italian seasoning	1 tbsp.
Sea salt	½ tsp.
Black pepper	½ tsp.
Chicken broth	1 cup

Cooking procedure:

1. First, place the chicken into the instant pot and add the Italian seasoning and the salt and pepper. Season well.
2. Now, pour the broth over the chicken. Close the lid and set the time to 10 minutes in high pressure.
3. Remove the chicken from the cooker and shred using two forks.
4. Serve with the broth.

Mouthwatering Chicken Breasts with Lemon

Overall cooking time: 10 min

Servings: 4

Nutrition info: Calories: 102, fat: 1.5g, Carbs: 0.6g, protein: 23g, sodium: 0.5g.

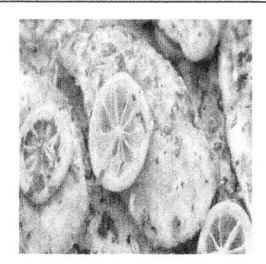

Ingredients:

Boneless chicken breasts	4
Chicken stock	4 cups
Lemon	1, thinly sliced
Thyme	4 springs
Peppercorns	1 tbsp.

Cooking procedure:

1. Add all the ingredients to the instant pot.
2. Close the lid and manually set the time to 5 minutes at high pressure.
3. When done, use natural pressure release for 2 minutes and then release the pressure and your dinner is ready.

Mojo Chicken

Overall cooking time: 45 min

Servings: 4

Nutrition info: Calories: 250, fat: 31g, Carbs: 1g, protein: 30g, sodium: 0.7g.

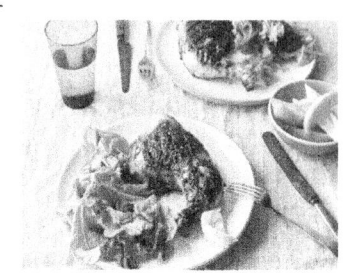

Ingredients:

Whole chicken	1
Olive oil	1 tbsp.
Lemon juice	1 tbsp.
Rosemary	2 tbsp.
Thyme	1 tbsp.
Sea salt	1 tbsp.
Black pepper	½ tbsp.
Bay leaf	1

Cooking procedure:

1. Switch the pressure cooker on to sauté and add the olive oil to the metal pan. Add the chicken and sauté both sides. Set aside.
2. Place the trivet and add the chicken stock, the lemon juice, rosemary, and thyme. Sprinkle the salt and pepper over the chicken.
3. Close the lid and press the button for poultry and cook for 25 to 30 minutes. Remove the chicken from the cooker and allow cooling before serving with bay leaf.

Spicy Chicken Curry with Coconut

Overall cooking time: 45 min

Servings: 4

Nutrition info: Calories: 472, fat: 25g, Carbs: 5g, protein: 57g, sodium: 245g.

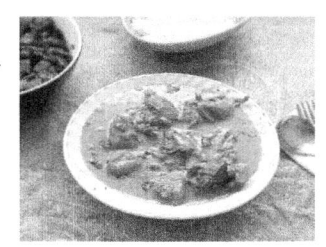

Ingredients:

Chicken breasts, boneless	3
Olive oil	2 tbsp.
Potatoes	4
Greek yogurt	½ cup
Coconut milk	1 cup

Spices

Fenugreek leaves	3 tbsp.
Coriander	1 tbsp.
Red chili	1 tbsp.
Turmeric powder	1 tbsp.
Cumin powder	1 tbsp.
Garlic	6 cloves
Ginger	1 tbsp.
Nutmeg	1 tbsp.
Cinnamon sticks	1
Bay leaves	1

Cooking procedure:

1. First, ready your spice items by cutting the main ingredients into small pieces.
2. Switch your instant pot to sauté temperature. Add the olive oil and all other spice ingredients. Sauté for 4 to 5 minutes. Add the chicken and sauté for another 5 minutes, to allow brown on both sides.
3. Now add the water, yogurt, coconut milk, garlic, tomatoes, and heat up to boil for 15 minutes.
4. Add the chopped potatoes, close the lid, and cook for 10 minutes at high pressure.

Quick All-in-one with Chicken and Rice

Overall cooking time: 30-40 min

Servings: 6

Nutrition info: Calories: 393, fat: 11 Carbs: 44g, protein: 30g, sugar: 3g.

Ingredients:

Onion	1 medium
Garlic	3 cloves
Baby carrots	2 cups.
Mushrooms	2 cups
Brown rice	2 cups
Olive oil	1 tbsp.
Chicken broth	2 ¼ cup
Chicken thigh	2 lbs.
Salt	1/8 tsp.
Black pepper	1/8 tsp.
Cream of chicken	10 oz.
Thyme	1 tbsp.

Cooking procedure:

1. Switch the pressure cooker to sauté and add the olive oil to the metal pan. Add the onion and sauté for 4 minutes.
2. Now add the broth, rice, garlic and veggies into the pot and mix. Then arrange the chicken on top. Sprinkle the salt and pepper over the chicken. Add the cream of chicken soup, the sprigs of thyme and close the lid.
3. Set the time to 30 minutes manually at high pressure.
4. Serve. You can shred the chicken too.

Beef Recipes

Mouthwatering Garlic Meatballs

Overall cooking time: 45 min

Servings: 4

Nutrition info: Calories: 192, fat: 11g, Carbs: 3g, protein: 32g, sodium: 0.06g.

Ingredients:

Ground beef	1 lb.
Spinach	1 cup
Garlic	¼ cup
Salt and pepper	to taste
Large carrot	4
Bone broth	as required

Cooking procedure:

1. First, chop the carrot into ½ inch chunks.
2. Add the chunks and the bone broth to an instant pot. In a large mixing bowl mix the beef with salt, pepper, garlic, and spinach and then roll up into convenient size meatballs.
3. Arrange the meatballs on the carrots chunks. Close the lid and manually set the time for 20 minutes at high pressure.
4. When the cooking is done, release the pressure and serve immediately.

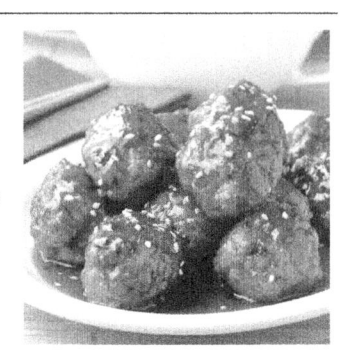

Homemade Spaghetti Squash and Meat Sauce

Overall cooking time: 30 min

Servings: 5

Nutrition info: Calories: 341, fat: 12g, Carbs: 17g, protein: 24g, sodium: 672mg.

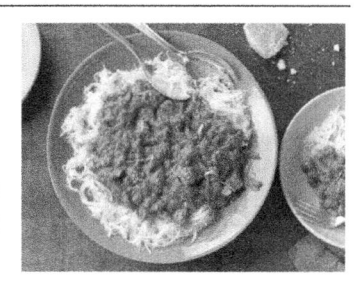

Ingredients:

Ground beef	1 lb.
Onion	1 small
Garlic cloves	3
Kosher salt	1 tbsp.
Black pepper	to taste
Tomatoes	8, crushed.
Bay leaf	as required
Spaghetti squash	1 large
Cheese	for topping

Cooking procedure:

1. Place the beef in the pot and add the salt, pepper, garlic, and onion. Set the cooker to sauté for 5 minutes. Add the crushed tomatoes, bay leaf, and cheese then stir.
2. Now take the spaghetti squash and pierce with a knife and place over the sauce. Close the lid and cook for 15 minutes.
3. When cooled, cut the spaghetti squash in half and scoop out the strands.
4. Serve squash with sauce and cheese.

Healthy Corned Beef

Overall cooking time: 55 min

Servings: 6

Nutrition info: Calories: 228, fat: 16g, Carbs: 3g, protein: 16g, sodium: 1g.

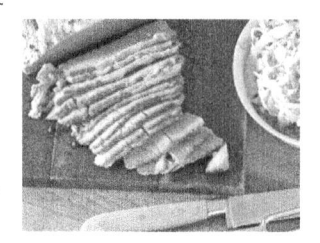

Ingredients:

Corned beef brisket	2 ½ lbs.
Red potatoes	20
Onion	1 medium
Garlic	cloves
Beef broth	4 cups.
Cabbage	1 head
Spice packet	1
Cornstarch	2 tbsp. (for gravy)

Cooking procedure:

1. Place the beef into the instant pot, add the garlic, potatoes, onion and pour the broth over everything. Sprinkle the spices over the whole arrangement.
2. Close the lid and set the time to 40 minutes at low pressure. After cooking, remove the lid and cool.
3. Now add the cabbage and cook again for 10 minutes. Remove the meat but not the drippings. Add 2 tbsp. cornstarch with the drippings.
4. Blend and cook until boiling. Lower the temperature and thicken slowly.

Easy Korean Beef

Overall cooking time: 45 min

Servings: 4

Nutrition info: Calories: 280, fat: 13g, Carbs: 15g, protein: 23g, sodium: 0.6g.

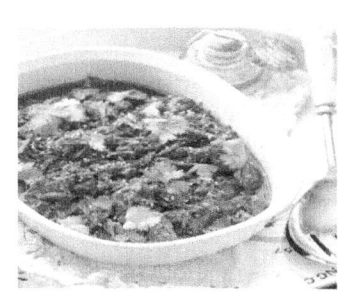

Ingredients:

Sesame oil	2 tbsp.
Lean beef	1 lb.
Garlic	1 clove
Brown sugar	¼ cup
Sodium soy sauce	¼ cup
Ground ginger	¼ tsp.
Red pepper	¼ tsp.
Green onion	1, sliced

Cooking procedure:

1. Set the instant pot's temperature to sauté and add the sesame oil. Add the beef with garlic and cook for 45 minutes.
2. Now add the soy sauce, ground ginger, red pepper and sugar. Combine well.
3. Close the lid and manually set the time to 5 minutes at high pressure.
4. After cooking, release the pressure and serve hot.

Delicious Braised Short Ribs

Overall cooking time: 45 min

Servings: 8

Nutrition info: Calories: 340, fat: 19g, Carbs: 8g, protein: 22g, sodium: 255mg.

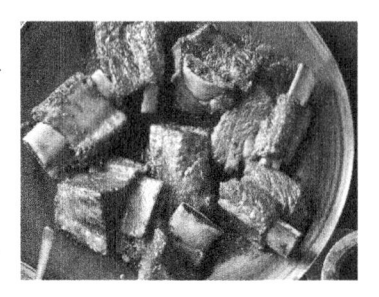

Ingredients:

Beef short ribs	4 lbs.
Kosher salt	1 pinch
Beef fat	1 tbsp.
Onion	1, quartered
Garlic	3 cloves
Water	1 cup

Cooking procedure:

1. Set the instant pot to the sauté temperature and spread the fat across the bottom. When it is heated, add the beef and sauté for 5 minutes.
2. Now add the garlic, onion, 1 cup water, c;ose the lid and cook for 35 minutes.
3. When cooking is done, serve on the bone or pull meat from bones.
4. Serve with rice or as you like most.

Healthy Beef with Broccoli

Overall cooking time: 50 min

Servings: 6

Nutrition info: Calories: 340, fat: 18g, Carbs: 38g, protein: 20g, sodium: 405mg.

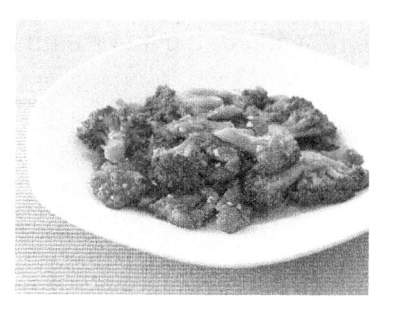

Ingredients:

Beef chuck roast	½ lbs.
Salt and pepper	½ tbsp.
Olive oil	2 tbsp.
Onion	1, chopped
Garlic cloves	4, minced
Beef broth	¾ cup
Soy sauce	½ cup
Brown sugar	1/3 cup
Sesame oil	2 tbsp.
Red pepper	1/8 tsp.
Broccoli florets	1 lb.
Water	3 tbsp.
Cornstarch	3 tbsp.

Cooking procedure:

1. Heat your instant pot to the sauté temperature and add olive oil into the hot pan. Season beef with pepper and salt. Set aside.
2. Add the onion to the pot and sauté for 2 minutes. Then add the garlic and sauté for 1 minute.
3. Now add red pepper, sesame oil, brown sugar, soy sauce and beef broth and stir until the sugar dissolves.
4. Add the beef and close the lid. Set the time for 12 minutes at high pressure.
5. Meanwhile, put the broccoli into a microwave with ¼ cup water and cook until tender.

6. In a mixing cup, mix the cornstarch with water and add to the instant pot. Add the broccoli too. Cook for 5 minutes more without the lid or until you like.

Delicious Beef Stroganoff

Overall cooking time: 27 min

Servings: 6-8

Nutrition info: Calories: 335, fat:8g Carbs: 22g, protein: 20g, sodium: 794mg.

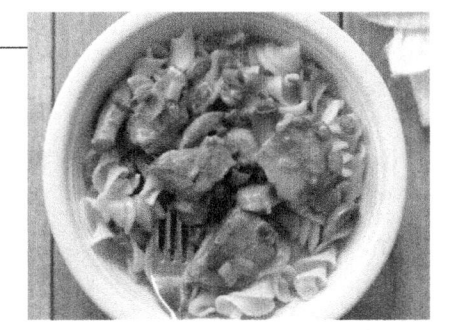

Ingredients:

EVOO	2 tbsp.	Mushrooms	3 cups, chopped
Onion	1/2, sliced	Flour	2 tbsp.
Bacon	1 piece, chopped	Beef broth	2 tbsp.
Salt	2 tbsp.	Chicken broth	2 cups
Ground pepper	1 tbsp.	Wide egg noodles	8oz.
Sirloin roast	1 lb.	Heavy cream	½ cup
Dried thyme	½ tsp.		

Cooking procedure:

1. Turn the instant pot to the sauté temperature and add the olive oil first. When heated, add the bacon, onion, and salt and sauté for 2-3 minutes. Add the roast pieces and season for 2 minutes more.
2. Add the meat and brown it with the onion and bacon. Now add the garlic, mushrooms, flour and then both broths.
3. Now add the egg noodles and the remaining ingredients except for the cream and spinach. Close the lid and cook for 17 minutes at high pressure.
4. When cooking is done, back to sauté, add the cream, and stir for 5 minutes.
5. Remove from the instant pot and mix with spinach.

Easy Mongolian Beef

Overall cooking time: 20 min

Servings: 6

Nutrition info: Calories: 370, fat: 6g, Carbs: 36g, protein: 38g, sodium: 523mg.

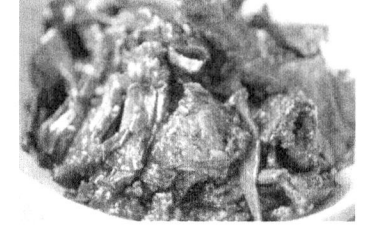

Ingredients:

Flank steak	2 lbs.
Vegetable oil	1 tbsp.
Garlic	4 cloves
Soy sauce	½ cup
Water	½ cup
Brown sugar	2/3 cup
Ginger	½ tsp., minced
Cornstarch	2 tbsp.
Onion	3, chopped

Cooking procedure:

1. Set the instant pot to sauté and season beef with pepper and salt. Set aside.
2. Add the garlic and sauté for 1 minute then add the soy sauce, ginger, brown sugar and ½ cup water. Stir to mix properly.
3. Now add the browned beef and the juices. Turn the instant pot to high pressure and set the time to 12 minutes.
4. Release the pressure and open the lid. Add the cornstarch and 3 tbsp. of water. Stir continuously and bring the temperature to a boil. Thicken until you're satisfied.

Delicious Beef Stew

Overall cooking time: 1 hour 15 min

Servings: 8

Nutrition info: Calories: 310, fat: 14g, Carbs: 26g, protein: 3.8g, sodium: 514mg.

Ingredients:

Chuck roast	2.5 lbs.
Vegetable oil	2 tbsp.
Kosher salt	1 tbsp.
Chicken stock	16oz.
Tomato sauce	16oz.
Potatoes	2 lbs. bite sized
Carrot	8oz. bite sized
Onion	2 large
Garlic	½ tsp.

Cooking procedure:

1. Set the instant pot to the sauté temperature and add the vegetable oil. When heated, add the bite-sized roast and sauté for 5 minutes.
2. Add the chicken stock and tomato sauce. Set the timer for 30 minutes at high pressure.
3. After cooking, open the lid and add the garlic powder, vegetables, and smoked paprika. Cook for 4 minutes manually.

Beef Bourguignon

Overall cooking time: 55 min

Servings: 4

Nutrition info: Calories: 440, fat: 17g, Carbs: 18g, protein: 42g, sodium: 1.03g.

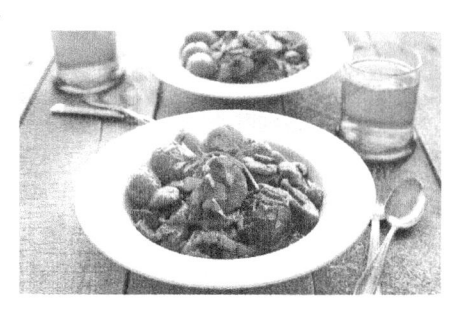

Ingredients:

Flank steak	1 lb.
Bacon	½ lb.
Carrots	5, cut into sticks
Garlic	2 cloves
Salt	2 tbsp.
Thyme	2 tbsp.
Parsley	2 tbsp.
Pepper	2 tbsp.
Red wine	1 cup
Beef broth	½ cup
Avocado oil	1 tbsp.
Sweet potato	2 large, cubed
Maple syrup	1 tbsp.

Cooking procedure:

1. Set the instant pot to the sauté and add the oil and heat. Add the beef and brown, stirring continually. Transfer.
2. Now add the bacon strips and onion. Brown and add the remaining ingredients.
3. Manually set the time for 30 minutes at high pressure and cook.
4. Yap, it's ready.

Red Wine Braised Beef Stew

Overall cooking time: 60 min

Servings: 8

Nutrition info: Calories: 232, fat: 10g, Carbs: 8g, protein: 20g, sodium: 215mg.

Ingredients:

Chuck roast	2 lbs.
Salt and pepper	a pinch
Gluten free flour	2 tbsp.
Olive oil	2 tbsp.
Onion	1, chopped
Garlic	3 cloves
Red wine	¾ cup
Tomato paste	1 tbsp.
Beef stock	½ cup
Thyme leaves	1 tbsp.
Bay leaves	2
Carrot	4, chopped

Cooking procedure:

1. Set the instant pot to sauté and season the beef with the sprinkle of flour and salt and pepper. Brown both sides.
2. Remove the beef from the instant pot and add the onion with 2 tbsp. of olive oil. Add the garlic and cook for another 30 seconds.
3. Now add the wine, tomato paste and stir to mix. Add the remaining ingredients to the browned beef.
4. Close the lid and manually set the time for 40 minutes at high pressure. Done.

Special Beef with Vegetables and Rice

Overall cooking time: 15 min

Servings: 4

Nutrition info: Calories: 190, fat: 2g, Carbs: 28g, protein: 6g, sodium: 0mg.

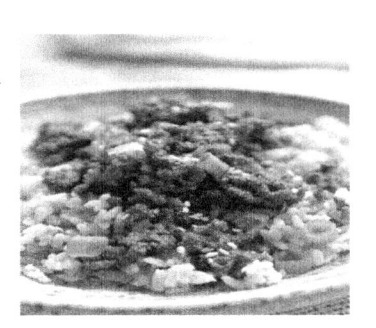

Ingredients:

Lean beef	1 lb.
Garlic	1 clove
Brown sugar	¼ cup
Soy sauce	¼ cup
Sesame oil	2 tbsp.
Ground ginger	¼ tsp.
Red pepper	¼ tsp.
Cooked rice	2 cups
Onion	3, sliced

Cooking procedure:

1. Before cooking, season your beef with everything except the oil and onion allow sitting for 2-3 hours.
2. Turn on your instant pot and set to sauté. Add the oil and heat. Add the meat and sauté for 5 minutes.
3. Now close the lid and set the time for 5 minutes at high pressure.
4. Transfer the meat to natural depressurization.

Healthy Pot Roast

Overall cooking time: 1 hour and 20 minutes.

Servings: 8

Nutrition info: Calories: 240, fat: 19g, Carbs: 2g, protein: 25g, sodium: 345mg.

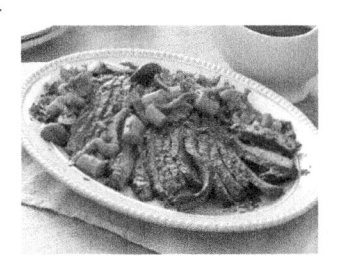

Ingredients:

Beef chuck	3 lbs.
Vegetable oil	1 tbsp.
Onion	1, chopped
Beef broth	1 cup
Bay leaves	2
Lemon peper	

Cooking procedure:

1. Season the roast with lemon pepper and set aside.
2. Set the instant pot to sauté and place the oil into it. When the oil is heated, add the meat and brown both sides. Remove the meat from the pot.
3. Now add the onion, water and bay leaves. Place the meat on top of the onion. Set the time for 70 minutes at high pressure.
4. Remove the lid and thicken as you want.

French Dip Sandwiches

Overall cooking time: 2 hours 30 minutes.

Servings: 6

Nutrition info: Calories: 740, fat: 41g, Carbs: 48g, protein: 35g, sodium: 1450mg.

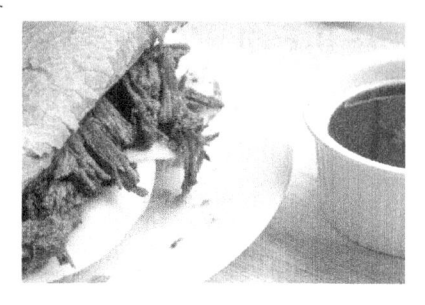

Ingredients:

Chuck roast	2.5 lbs.	Beef broth	1 14oz
Vegetable oil	1 tbsp.	Bay leaf	1
Kosher salt	2 tbsp.	Soft rolls	6
Ground pepper	to taste	Butter	3 tbsp.
Garlic powder	½ tsp.	Salt	1 pinch
Onion	1, sliced	Provolone cheese	6 slices
Red wine	½ cup		

Cooking procedure:

1. Add the vegetable oil to the instant pot and heat the pot to sauté.
2. Season the meat with salt, pepper, and garlic on all sides.
3. In your instant pot, sear the roast using two kitchen tongs and set aside.
4. Add the onion to the instant pot and sauté for 3 minutes. Add the red wine and bring the heat to boil. Then lower the heat, add the broth and the bay leaf and then add the roast into the instant pot.
5. Close the lid and set the time to 100 minutes at high pressure. Now remove the lid, transfer the meat to a serving plate and shred.

6. Broil the sandwich rolls in the oven and mix the butter with garlic powder and salt. Brush the rolls with this mixture and toast for 3 minutes.
7. Pile the shred meat onto the rolls and top with cheese. Heat to melt the cheese.
8. Top sandwich with parsley and serve with dipping sauce.

Cheeseburger Macaroni

Overall cooking time: 25 min

Servings: 4

Nutrition info: Calories: 340, fat: 17g, Carbs: 28g, protein: 22g, sodium: 0.8mg.

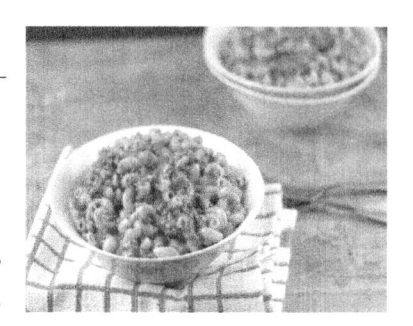

Ingredients:

Vegetable oil	1 tbsp.
Lean beef	1 lb.
Yellow onion	1, diced
Salt	½ tbsp.
Pepper	½ tbsp.
Thyme	12 tbsp.
Ketchup	¼ cup
Elbow macaroni	3 cups
Beef stock	3 cups
Velveeta cheese	12 oz.

Cooking procedure:

1. Brown the beef first with a little oil.
2. Add all the ingredients except the cheese and close the lid. Set the time for 8 minutes at high pressure.
3. Quickly release the pressure, open the lid and add the cheese. Stir until it becomes creamy.
4. Leave it for 5 minutes.

Pork, Turkey and Lamb Recipes

Instant Pulled Pork

Overall cooking time: 1hrs and 35 min

Servings: 8

Nutrition info: Calories: 240, fat: 5.8g, Carbs: 18g, protein: 26g, sodium: 655mg.

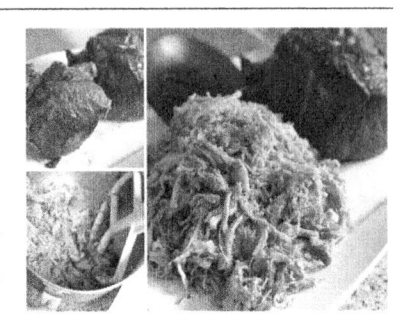

Ingredients:

Pork shoulder	2 lbs.
Onion powder	1 tbsp.
Garlic powder	1 tbsp.
Mustard powder	1 tbsp.
Salt	2 tsp.
Pepper	½ tbsp.
BBQ sauce	½ cup
Water	½ cup

Cooking procedure:

1. In a large mixing bowl, mix all the dry ingredients together. Take the pork and rub it with the mixture.
2. Place the pork into the instant pot and add the BBQ sauce. Close the lid and cook for 1 hour at high pressure.
3. When the cooking is done, shred the meat using two forks.
4. Add more BBQ sauce at the top of your serving plate.

Dr. Pepper Pulled Pork

Overall cooking time: 52 min

Servings: 4

Nutrition info: Calories: 206, fat: 5.5g, Carbs: 12g, protein: 26g, sodium: 550mg.

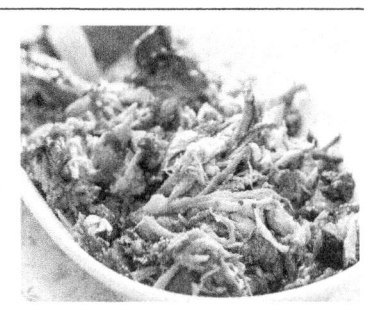

Ingredients:

Dr. Pepper	2 cups
BBQ sauce	1 cup
Pork roast	4 lbs.
Onion powder	1 tbsp.
Garlic powder	1 tbsp.
Salt	1 tsp.

Cooking procedure:

1. First, cut the pork into three or four chunks. In a large mixing bowl, mix the onion powder, garlic powder, and salt and fold the meat chunks with it.
2. Put the pork into the instant pot, add the Dr. Pepper and the BBQ sauce.
3. Fasten the lid and set the time to 50 minutes at high pressure.
4. After cooking, release the pressure and drain the liquid from the meat. Separate the meat to a serving plate and shred using two forks.
5. Enjoy your favorite sauce.

Easy Instant BBQ Ribs

Overall cooking time: 41 min

Servings: 3

Nutrition info: Calories: 340, fat: 19g, Carbs: 8g, protein: 22g, sodium: 255mg.

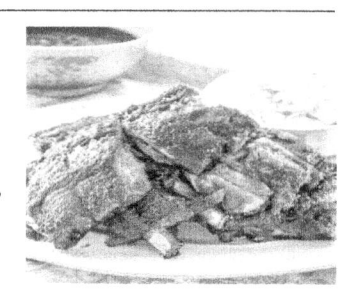

Ingredients:

Baby back ribs	1 rack
BBQ sauce	4 tbsp.
Salt	¼ tsp.
Black pepper	¼ tsp.
Liquid smoke	a few drop

Cooking procedure:

1. First, remove the membrane from the ribs with a towel and then season with salt and pepper.
2. Take your instant pot, add 1 cup of water and set the trivet inside. Now place the ribs on the trivet and close the lid. Set the time for 20 minutes at high pressure.
3. Release the pressure, open the lid and remove the ribs.
4. Apply the BBQ sauce with a brush all over the ribs and arrange on a baking tray. Transfer them to the oven for 10 to 15 minutes at 450 F.

Delicious Rich Creamy Pork Chops

Overall cooking time: 30 min

Servings: 3-6

Nutrition info: Calories: 667, fat:29g, Carbs: 10g, protein: 52g, sodium: 755mg.

Ingredients:

Pork chops	6
Pepper	¼ tsp.
Oil	2-3 tbsp.
Water	1 ½ cups
Mushroom soup	10 oz.
Sour cream	1 ½ cups
Fresh parsley	1 tbsp.

Cooking procedure:

1. Set the instant pot to sauté temperature and add the oil. When heated, add the pork and sauté for 5 minutes on both sides.
2. Add water and then add the chops to the pot again.
3. Close the lid and cook for 8 minutes. Separate the chops and keep warm.
4. Now, whisk the chops into the sour cream and heat a little but do not boil.
5. At the end, stir in parsley.

Tex-Mex Chili Mac

Overall cooking time: 25 min

Servings: 8

Nutrition info: Calories: 276, fat: 7g, Carbs: 30g, protein: 179g, sodium: 855mg.

Ingredients:

Vegetable oil	1 tbsp.
Lean ground sausage	1 lb.
Yellow onion	1, diced
Water	1 cup
Elbow macaroni	2 cups
Green chilies	1 can
Chili powder	1 tbsp.
Salt	1 tsp.
Cayenne pepper	¼ tsp.
Frozen Corn	1 cup
Fresh cilantro	2 tbsp.

Cooking procedure:

1. Set the instant pot to sauté and add the oil. When heated, add the meat with onion and garlic and sauté for 10 minutes.
2. Now add the water, green chilies, macaroni, chili powder, tomato sauce, cayenne pepper, and salt. Stir to combine all.
3. Set the time for 5 minutes at high pressure.
4. When the cooking is done, add the frozen corn and stir. Set the instant pot to sauté and cook to make the macaroni tender.
5. Now add the cilantro and stir to combine well.
6. Serve hot with sour cream, tortilla chips, and Mexican cheese.

Simple Pork Adobo

Overall cooking time: 30 min

Servings: 5-6

Nutrition info: Calories: 342, fat: 19g, Carbs: 2g, protein: 32g, sodium: 793mg.

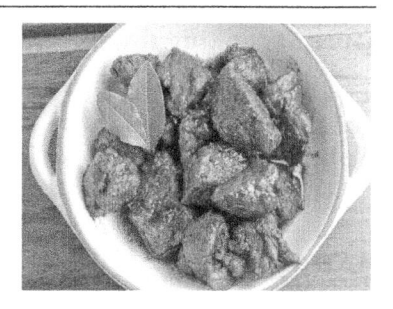

Ingredients:

Short ribs	2 lbs.
Garlic	6 cloves
Soy sauce	½ cup
Vinegar	1 cup
Peppercorn	1 tbsp.
Bay leaves	4
Salt and pepper	to taste
Corn starch	1 tbsp.

Cooking procedure:

1. Sauté the meat with oil and garlic. Add a pinch of salt and pepper when sautéing.
2. Now add the brown sugar and combine with the meat to blend properly. Add the vinegar, soy sauce, corn, black pepper and bay leaves. Mix.
3. Close the lid and set the time for 15 minutes at high pressure.
4. Turn to sauté again and add a mixture of water and cornstarch to the meat. Now bring the temperature to boil for 5 minutes.
5. Serve over cooked rice.

Amazing Pork Carnitas

Overall cooking time: 55 min

Servings: 6

Nutrition info: Calories: 200, fat: 14g, Carbs: 0g, protein: 20g.

Ingredients:

Pork shoulder	1 lb.
Onion	1/2, sliced
Garlic cloves	4
Dried oregano	1 tbsp.
Cumin	2 tsp.
Chili powder	1 tbsp.
Cinnamon	¼ tsp.
Bay leaf	1
Kosher salt	3 tsp.
Lime juice	for serving

Cooking procedure:

1. First, add the grapefruit juice to the instant pot.
2. Take a mixing bowl and add the meat chunks, garlic, grapefruit zest, salt, chili powder, cumin, and oregano. Combine.
3. Now add the meat, bay leaf, and onion to the instant pot. Close the lid and set the time for 35 minutes.
4. Preheat your oven and then transfer the meat from the cooker to a baking sheet.
5. Shred the meat and place in the oven. Brown the meat until a little brittle.
6. Serve with your favorite juice and cilantro.

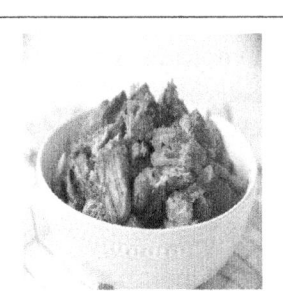

Quick and Easy Pork Chops

Overall cooking time: 25 min

Servings: 2

Nutrition info: Calories: 273, fat: 7g, Carbs: 4g, protein: 45g.

Ingredients:

Lemon pepper	2 tbsp.
Pork chops	2, boneless
Apple juice	¼ cup

Cooking procedure:

1. First, coat the chops with the lemon pepper.
2. Set your instant pot to sauté and brown the chops. Now, remove the chops from the cooker and add the apple juice at the surface of the chops. Then, place the chops in the instant pot and manually set the time to 10 minutes and cook.
3. At last, remove the chops again and sauté the sauce a little and serve.

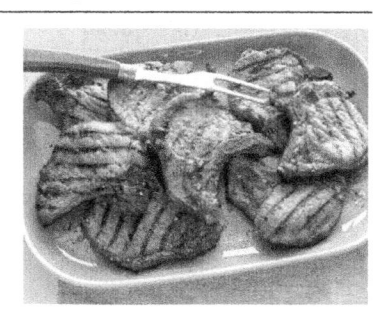

Instant Turkey Breast

Overall cooking time: 45 min

Servings: 7

Nutrition info: Calories: 120, fat: 1g, Carbs: 0g, protein: 28g.

Ingredients:

Turkey breast	6.5 lbs.
Salt and pepper	to taste
Chicken broth	14 oz.
Onion	1 large
Stock celery	1
Thyme	1 sprig
Cornstarch	3 tbsp.

Cooking procedure:

1. Mix the turkey with salt and pepper very well.
2. Place the trivet in the instant pot and add the celery, thyme, onion and chicken broth. Now add the turkey and set the time to 30 minutes at high pressure.
3. The turkey should cook completely, if not then cook for 3 to 5 minutes more.
4. In a mixing bowl, mix the cornstarch and a cup of water and add with the broth to the instant pot. Sauté to thicken the broth mixture.
5. Slice the turkey and serve.

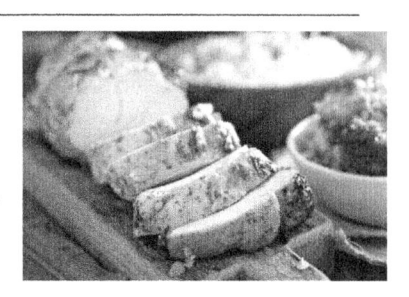

Mouthwatering DIY Sandwiches

Overall cooking time: 45 min

Servings: 5-6

Nutrition info: Calories: 220, fat: 2g, Carbs: 42g, protein: 8g.

Ingredients:

Turkey breast	2 lbs.
Seasoning	½ cup
Garlic	2 cloves
Avocado oil	1/3 cup
Chicken broth	1 cup

Cooking procedure:

1. First, season the turkey with the seasoning of your choice.
2. Set the instant pot to sauté and sauté the turkey on both sides.
3. Now, place the trivet and then pour the chicken broth into the pot and add the garlic. Set the time for 30 minutes.
4. Remove the turkey from the pot, cool and slice as you like most.

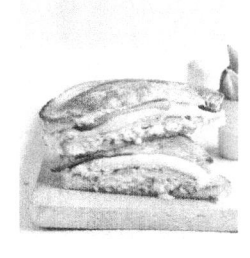

Homemade Cabbage Turkey Sausage

Overall cooking time: 15 min

Servings: 5

Nutrition info: Calories: 187, fat:9g, Carbs: 7g, protein: 17g.

Ingredients:

Turkey sausage	1lb
Cabbage	1 head
Onion	1, diced
Garlic	3 cloves
Sugar	2 tbsp.
Balsamic vinegar	2 tbsp.
Dijon mustard	2 tsp.
Olive oil	2 tbsp.
Salt and pepper	to taste

Cooking procedure:

1. Brown the sausage with onion and oil in your instant pot.
2. Now add the cabbage and the all other ingredients into the instant pot and set the temperature to sauté. Cook for 5-7 minutes.
3. Now test your dinner's taste, adjust with salt and pepper, as needed.

Healthy Turkey Verde & Rice

Overall cooking time: 30 min

Servings: 5

Nutrition info: Calories: 430 fat: 15g Carbs: 13g, protein: 29g.

Ingredients:

Chicken broth	2/3 cup
Brown rice	1 ¼ cup
Yellow onion	1 small
Salsa verde	½ cup
Jennie-O turkey tenderloins	1 ½ lbs.
Salt	½ tbsp.

Cooking procedure:

1. Add the chicken broth and rice to your instant pot. Also, add the onion, salsa verde, and the turkey. Sprinkle the salt and pepper to taste.
2. Now, close the lid and set the time to 18 minutes at high pressure. Then set aside for 10 minutes.
3. Top with fresh cilantro.

Delicious Lamb Stew

Overall cooking time: 1 hour 30 min

Servings: 4

Nutrition info: Calories: 378, fat: 15g Carbs: 24g, protein: 34g.

Ingredients:

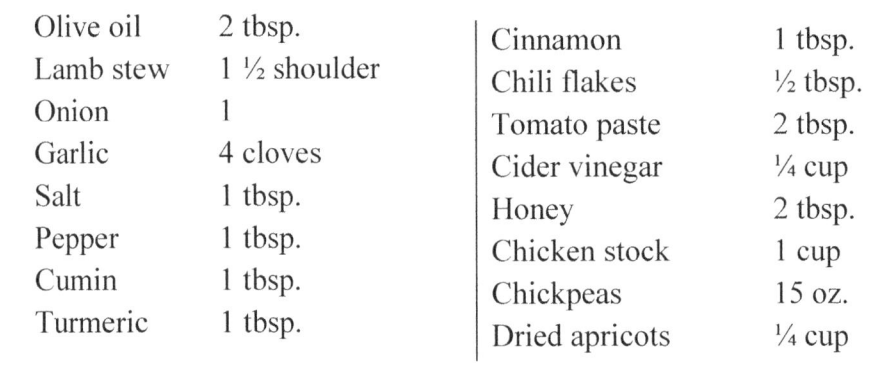

Olive oil	2 tbsp.	Cinnamon	1 tbsp.
Lamb stew	1 ½ shoulder	Chili flakes	½ tbsp.
Onion	1	Tomato paste	2 tbsp.
Garlic	4 cloves	Cider vinegar	¼ cup
Salt	1 tbsp.	Honey	2 tbsp.
Pepper	1 tbsp.	Chicken stock	1 cup
Cumin	1 tbsp.	Chickpeas	15 oz.
Turmeric	1 tbsp.	Dried apricots	¼ cup

Cooking procedure:

1. Turn your instant pot to sauté and heat the olive oil with onion for 3 minutes. Then add the lamb, salt, garlic and the other spices and sauté for 5 minutes more.
2. Close the lid and set the time to 1 hour without switching to the meat button.
3. Serve with rice and top with quinoa and parsley.

Super Easy Lamb Curry

Overall cooking time: 50 min

Servings: 6

Nutrition info: Calories: 335, fat: 22g, Carbs: 0.5g, protein: 28g.

Ingredients:

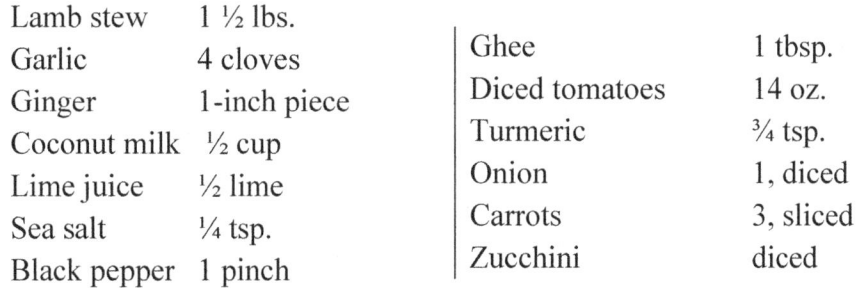

Lamb stew	1 ½ lbs.
Garlic	4 cloves
Ginger	1-inch piece
Coconut milk	½ cup
Lime juice	½ lime
Sea salt	¼ tsp.
Black pepper	1 pinch
Ghee	1 tbsp.
Diced tomatoes	14 oz.
Turmeric	¾ tsp.
Onion	1, diced
Carrots	3, sliced
Zucchini	diced

Cooking procedure:

1. In a large mixing bowl, mix the meat with garlic, ginger, lime, milk, pepper, and salt. Transfer the whole mixture to a refrigerator for marinating.
2. Place the marinated meat in the instant pot and add the tomatoes, ghee, masala, carrots, and onion. Seal the lid and set the time to 15 minutes at high pressure.
3. Release the pressure and set to sauté. Add the zucchini and cook for 5 to 6 minutes to permit the zucchini to tenderize.
4. Serve with rice.

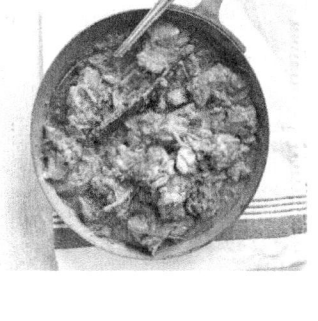

Lamb Rogan Josh

Overall cooking time: 30 min

Servings: 5-6

Nutrition info: Calories: 383, fat: 29g, Carbs: 11g, protein: 21g.

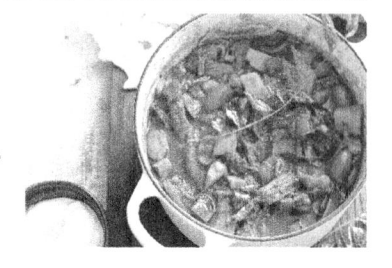

Ingredients:

Leg of lamb	1 ½ lbs	Fennel seeds	1 tbsp.
Greek yogurt	4 tbsp.	Garlic	2 cloves
Masala	½ tbsp.	Garam masala	½ tbsp.
Olive oil	1 tbsp.	Ground chili	½ tbsp.
Bay leaves	2	Coriander	1 tbsp.
Cardamom pods	3	Ginger	1 tbsp.
Cinnamon bark	2-inch	Tomatoes	2
Whole cloves	2	Coriander	1 tbsp.
Cumin seeds	1 ½ tbsp.	Salt and pepper	to taste.

Cooking procedure:

1. In a mixing bowl, mix the lamb with garam masala and yogurt. Marinate the mixture in the refrigerator for 24 hours.
2. Now, set the instant pot to sauté and add the oil. After 2 minutes, add the spice items, except for the powder ingredients and sauté for 3 minutes. Add the garlic and remaining powder ingredients. During the last of sautéing, add the tomato and a cup of water.
3. Then add the marinated lamb and stir evenly. Close the lid and manually set the time to 10 minutes.
4. Remove the lid and set back to sauté. Stir and cook to your desired tenderness. Add a little salt and pepper if needed.
5. Cook rice to serve with it.

Vegetable Recipes

Veggie Cauli Rice

Overall cooking time: 20 min

Servings: 4

Nutrition info: Calories: 260, fat: 13g, Carbs: 28g, protein: 8g.

Ingredients:

Head of cauliflower	1 medium
Olive oil	2 tbsp.
Salt	¼ tbsp.
Parsley	½ tsp.
Seasoning	1 tbsp.
Paprika	¼ tbsp.
Cilantro	as required
Lime juice	½ tbsp.

Cooking procedure:

1. Take the cauliflower and trim off the leaves. Wash thoroughly and chop it into few pieces.
2. Place the pieces into the instant pot with a cup of water. Close the lid. Manually set the time for 2 minutes. It will first take 10 minutes to develop the pressure.
3. When it is done, remove the cauliflower and set aside.
4. Remove any extra water from the pot and bring the cooker to sauté. Add the oil and then the cauliflower. Break up the flower with the help of a potato masher.
5. Now add the spice ingredients with salt and pepper.
6. Serve with sauces or with other dishes.

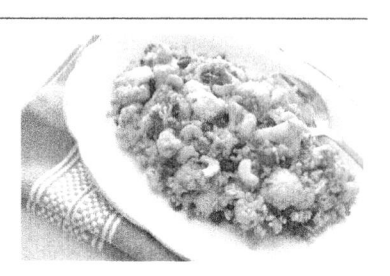

Delicious Lentils in the Instant Pot

Overall cooking time: 30 min

Servings: 3

Nutrition info: Calories: 237, fat: 1.9g, Carbs: 42g, protein: 15g.

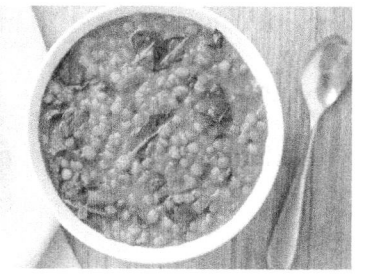

Ingredients:

Lentils	1 cup
Onion	½ cup, chopped
Garlic	2 cloves, minced
Chili powder	½ tbsp.
Cumin	¼ tbsp.
Jalapeno	½, diced
Olive oil	1 tbsp.
Water	1 ¼ cups
Sea salt	½ tbsp.

Cooking procedure:

1. Take a large bowl and add the lentils. Rinse thoroughly. Pour enough water to just cover the lentils. Leave for several hours.
2. Drain the water and put them into the instant pot. Add the other ingredients.
3. Close the lid and set on the chili button. Manually set the time for 7 minutes.
4. Serve over rice.

Curried Peas Curry

Overall cooking time: 20 min

Servings: 5-6

Nutrition info: Calories: 130, fat: 0.7g, Carbs: 18.5g, protein: 7g.

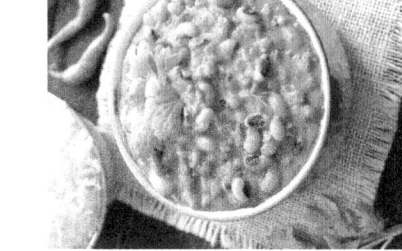

Ingredients:

Black-eyed peas	1 lb.
Onion	1, chopped
Garlic	4 cloves, minced
Ginger	2 tbsp.
Turmeric	2 tbsp.
Cumin	1 tbsp.
Coriander	1 tbsp.
Cayenne	1/16 tsp.
Sea salt	1 ½ tsp.

Cooking procedure:

1. Take a large bowl and add the dried peas. Rinse and soak the peas for several hours.
2. Now drain the water, add the peas into the instant pot, and then add the onion and 2 cups of water. Add the all other ingredients.
3. Close the lid and press the Bean button for 3 minutes.
4. Add a pinch of salt if required and adjust the seasoning.
5. Serve over cooked rice with cilantro leaves.

Simple Pinto Beans

Overall cooking time: 20 min

Servings: 8

Nutrition info: Calories: 230, fat: 10g, Carbs: 25g, protein: 10g.

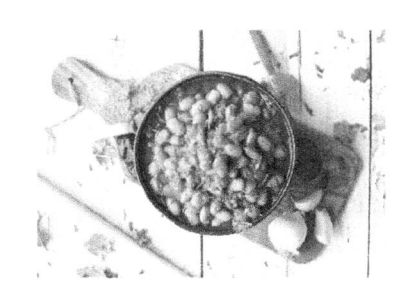

Ingredients:

Pinto beans	1lb.
Onion	1, chopped
Garlic	4 cloves, minced
Pepper	1
Tomato	½, chopped
Chili powder	1 tbsp.
Cumin	2 tbsp.
Oregano	1 ½ tbsp.
Sea salt	1 ¼ tsp.

Cooking procedure:

1. Take a large bowl and add the beans. Rinse thoroughly. Cover with water to soak and leave for several hours.
2. Now, drain the water and put the beans in the pot with the remaining ingredients. Stir to mix.
3. Close the lid and cook using the chili function for 22 minutes. Allow to depressurize naturally.
4. Serve with cilantro leaves.

Healthy Brussels Sprouts

Overall cooking time: 18 min

Servings: 4

Nutrition info: Calories: 67, fat: 5g, Carbs: 5.2g, protein: 2g.

Ingredients:

Brussels sprouts	1lb.
Olive oil	2 tbsp.
Salt and pepper	1 pinch each
Pine nuts	¼ cup

Cooking procedure:

1. First, take your instant pot trivet, set inside the pot, and then place the steamer basket.
2. Add one cup of water and then the Brussels sprouts.
3. Fasten the lid and set the time to 3 minutes at high pressure.
4. Season with pine nuts, salt, pepper, olive oil, etc.

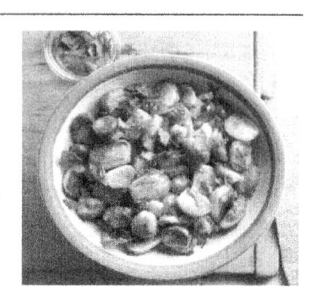

Super Simple & Sweet Brussels Sprouts

Overall cooking time: 15 min

Servings: 8

Nutrition info: Calories: 65, fat: 0g, Carbs: 3g, protein: n/a.

Ingredients:

Brussels sprouts	2 lbs.
Orange juice	¼ cup
Orange zest	1 tsp.
Buttery spread	1 tbsp.
Maple syrup	2 tbsp.
Black pepper	¼ tsp.
Salt	½ tbsp.

Cooking procedure:

1. Place all of the ingredients in the Instant Pot. First, making sure that the quick release switch is closed.
2. Then push the manual button and set the time for 3 to 4 minutes, but first cut the Brussels sprouts into small pieces. (You can always cook them longer if they aren't done to your liking by just setting the lid back over the pot and letting them sit in the pot a minute or two more.)
3. When the time is up, hit the off button and quick release the pressure.
4. Stir until the Brussels sprouts are evenly covered with sauce and serve.

Easy Baked Potato

Overall cooking time: 30 min

Servings: 5-6

Nutrition info: Calories: 161, fat: 0.2g, Carbs: 32g, protein: 4.5g.

Ingredients:

Potatoes   2lbs or however many you want

Cooking procedure:

1. Take your instant pot and place the steamer rack into it. Add the potatoes and then pour in one cup of water.
2. Close the lid and manually set the time for 10 minutes.
3. Remove the potatoes and eat.

Delicious Mashed Potatoes with Rosemary

Overall cooking time: 30 min

Servings: 5-6

Nutrition info: Calories: 108, fat: 4.5g, Carbs: 15g, protein: 2g.

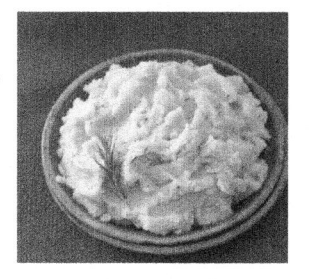

Ingredients:

Potatoes	6, peeled and cubed
Chicken broth	1 cup
Garlic	3 cloves
Rosemary	1 sprig
Butter	2 tbsp.
Milk	¼ cup

Cooking procedure:

1. Place the potatoes into the instant pot and add the garlic, chicken broth, butter and rosemary sprig.
2. Close the lid and set the time for 15 minutes. Then quickly release the pressure.
3. Separate the potatoes and mash them with milk and butter to make them creamy and smooth.
4. You will like it.

Quick Mango Mashed Potatoes

Overall cooking time: 11 min

Servings: 6

Nutrition info: Calories: 142, fat: 1.9g, Carbs: 7g, protein: 54g.

Ingredients:

Potatoes	2 lbs.
Water	1 cup
Butter	½ stick
Milk	1 cup
Salt and pepper	to taste
Mango juice	½ cup

Cooking procedure:

1. Place all ingredients except the mango juice and milk into the instant pot.
2. Secure the lid and set the time for 7 minutes.
3. Open the lid and separate the potatoes into a large mixing bowl. Mash the potatoes with milk and mango juice until they become soft and even in color.
4. Enjoy your dish.

Mushrooms with Green Beans and Bacon

Overall cooking time: 30 min

Servings: 5

Nutrition info: Calories: 120, fat: 5g, Carbs: 7g, protein: 5g.

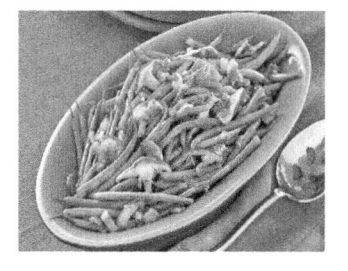

Ingredients:

Green beans	1 lb.
Bacon	6oz., chopped
Onion	1/2, sliced
Mushrooms	8oz., sliced
Garlic	1 clove
Balsamic vinegar	1 splash
Salt and pepper	to taste

Cooking procedure:

1. Place the green beans into the instant pot and pour a cup of water over them.
2. Close the lid and set the time for 2 minutes at high pressure.
3. Separate the green beans and drain the water. Set aside.
4. Now, turn the cooker to sauté and add the bacon and a little pepper, add the mushrooms and cook for several minutes stirring to make the bacon crispy.
5. Add the green beans back to the cooker and the vinegar. Stir to mix properly.
6. Season and enjoy.

Quick Asparagus Dinner

Overall cooking time: 10 min

Servings: 2-3

Nutrition info: Calories: 26.8, fat: .19g, Carbs: 5.2g, protein: 2.9g.

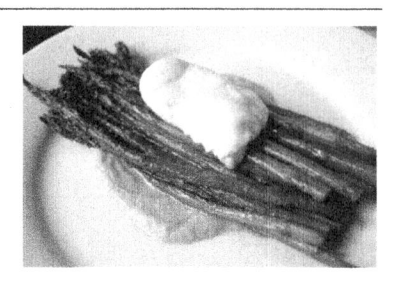

Ingredients:

Asparagus	1 lb.
Water	1 cup
Onion powder	1 tbsp.
Olive oil	2 tbsp.
Salt and pepper	to taste

Cooking procedure:

1. Take the steamer basket and place it into the instant pot.
2. Pour in the water and place the asparagus into the instant pot basket. Sprinkle the onion powder and drizzle the oil.
3. Now close the lid and manually set the time to 3 minutes.
4. Open the cover, separate on a serving plate and sprinkle with a little salt and pepper.

Delicious Mashed Sweet Potato

Overall cooking time: 25 min

Servings: 3

Nutrition info: Calories: 142, fat: 3g, Carbs: 27g, protein: 2g.

Ingredients:

Sweet potato	2 lbs.
Unsalted butter	3 tbsp.
Maple syrup	2 tbsp.
Nutmeg	¼ tsp.
Water	1 cup
Salt and pepper	to taste

Cooking procedure:

1. First, cut the peeled sweet potatoes into 1-inch chunks.
2. Add them to the instant pot and pour in a cup of water. Close the lid and set the time for 8 minutes.
3. When done, remove the cover and transfer the potatoes to a bowl. Add the butter and maple syrup and mash the potatoes. Sprinkle with a pinch of salt and pepper.

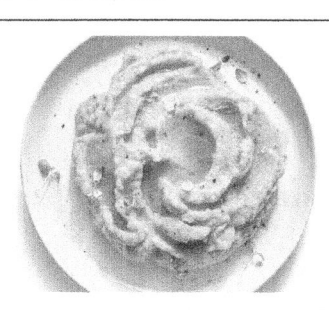

Simple Corn on the Cob

Overall cooking time: 20 min

Servings: 2

Nutrition info: Calories: 80, fat: 0.5g, Carbs: 20g, protein: 3g.

Ingredients:

Corn on the cob	1
Kosher salt	½ tbsp.
Water	1 cup
Butter	3 tbsp.

Cooking procedure:

1. Remove the silk and husks from the corn, then cut off the steam to the ends of the corn.
2. Arrange the ears into the instant pot, pour in the water, sprinkle the salt over the corn, and then add the butter.
3. Close the lid and set the time for 3 minutes.
4. Now, drain the corn so that the extra water drips back into the cooker and place it on a serving plate.
5. Serve with salt and butter.

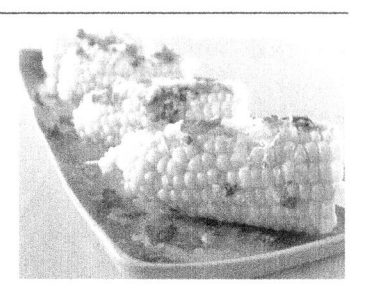

Delicious Pinto Bean Mash

Overall cooking time: 30 min

Servings: 4

Nutrition info: Calories: 110, fat: 1g, Carbs: 16g, protein: 6g.

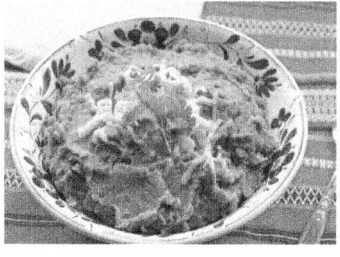

Ingredients:

Pinto beans	3 cups
Water	4 cups
Onion	1, quartered
Garlic	3 cloves
Red wine vinegar	3 tbsp.
Salt and pepper	to taste
Cumin	1 tbsp.

Cooking procedure:

1. Take a bowl and pour the beans into it. Add water to cover the beans and soak overnight.
2. Place the beans into the instant pot after draining the water. Add the garlic, onion, and 4 cups water.
3. Close the lid and set the time to 28 minutes at medium pressure.
4. After cooking, carefully release the pressure, open the lid, add the all other ingredients, and then mash evenly.
5. What? Enjoy.

Mouthwatering Smothered Cajun Greens

Overall cooking time: 35 min

Servings: 4

Nutrition info: Calories: 430, fat: 14g, Carbs: 20g, protein: 32g.

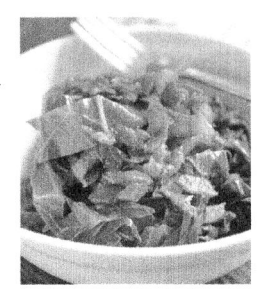

Ingredients:

Raw greens	6 cups
Turnip	1, chopped
Onion	1, chopped
Uncured ham	1 lb. cooked
Animal fat	1 tbsp.
Crushed garlic	2 tbsp.
Salt	to taste
Poultry broth	½ cup

Cooking procedure:

1. Put all the ingredients into the instant pot and close the lid. Manually set the time for 20 minutes at high pressure.
2. Turn off the cooker and naturally release the pressure.
3. Stir and serve.

Rice and Quinoa Recipes

Chipotle's Cilantro Lime Rice

Overall cooking time: 15 min

Servings: 6

Nutrition info: Calories: 118, fat: 10g, Carbs: 29g, protein: 5g.

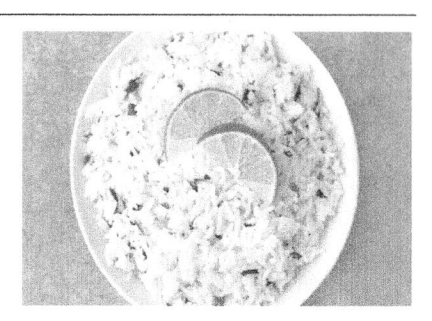

Ingredients:

White rice	1 cup
Water	1 1/4 cups
Vegetable oil	2 tbsp.
Salt	1 tsp.
Lime juice	1 tbsp.
Cilantro	3 tbsp.

Cooking procedure:

1. Place the rice, 1 tbsp. of olive oil, salt, and water into the instant pot. Stir to mix and then close the lid.
2. Set the time for 3 minutes at high pressure.
3. When the cooking is done, naturally release the pressure and then fluff the rice a little.
4. Now add the chopped cilantro, the rest of the oil and the lime juice. Mix and serve.

Delicious Coconut Lime Quinoa

Overall cooking time: 35 min

Servings: 6

Nutrition info: Calories: 341, fat: 20g, Carbs: 35g, protein: 7g.

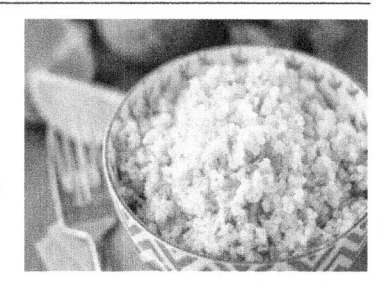

Ingredients:

Quinoa	1 cup
Coconut milk	14 oz.
Water	¼ cup
Salt	¼ tsp.
Small lime	1, zested and juiced

Cooking procedure:

1. Add all the ingredients except the lime juice into the instant pot and close the lid. Set the time for 30 minutes at low pressure.
2. When done, open the lid and fluff the rice.
3. Transfer the rice to a bowl and add the zest and juice. Stir with a sprinkle of salt.
4. It's ready.

Quick and Easy Quinoa

Overall cooking time: 35 min

Servings: 4

Nutrition info: Calories: 172, fat: 3g, Carbs: 31g, protein: 6g.

Ingredients:

Quinoa	1 cup
Water	1 ½ cups
Salt	1 pinch

Cooking procedure:

1. Pour the quinoa into the instant pot and add the water.
2. Close the lid and set the time for 1 minute at high pressure.
3. When cooking is over, open the pot with natural pressure release. Transfer the quinoa to a serving plate. Add a pinch of salt and stir.
4. Done.

Delicious Parmesan Risotto

Overall cooking time: 25 min

Servings: 8

Nutrition info: Calories: 247, fat: 5.1g, Carbs: 30g, protein: n/a.

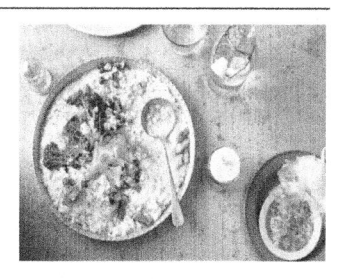

Ingredients:

Butter	2 tbsp.
Shallots	½ cup, chopped
Garlic	3 cloves
Grain rice	1 1/3 cups
White wine	1 cup
Chicken broth	3 cups
Cheese	2 oz.
Salt	to taste

Cooking procedure:

1. Turn your instant pot to sauté and add the butter. When the butter melts, add the shallots and sauté for 3 minutes.
2. Now add the garlic and sauté until fragrant. Add the rice and stir continuously to coat the rice with butter. Cook for 1 minute. Then add the white wine and stir evenly.
3. Add the broth and parmesan, half of the cheese and sprinkle a pinch of salt. Stir again.
4. Close the lid and set the time for 10 minutes at high pressure.
5. Add rest of the cheese and serve.

Easy Spanish Rice

Overall cooking time: 30 min

Servings: 8

Nutrition info: Calories: 98, fat: 4g, Carbs: 14g, protein: 1.3g.

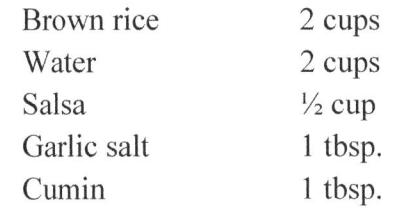

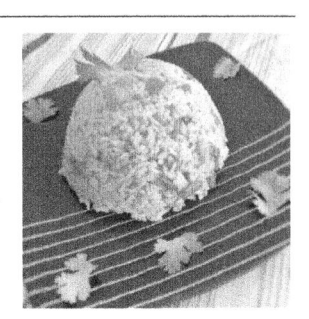

Ingredients:

Brown rice	2 cups
Water	2 cups
Salsa	½ cup
Garlic salt	1 tbsp.
Cumin	1 tbsp.

Cooking procedure:

1. Put all the ingredients into the instant pot and close the lid. Manually set the time for 22 minutes at high pressure. Allow cooking.
2. Turn off the cooker and naturally release the pressure.
3. Fluff and serve.

Dessert Recipes

Delicious Vanilla Bean Cheesecake

Overall cooking time: 25 min

Servings: 8

Nutrition info: Calories: 273, fat: 14g, Carbs: 24g, protein: 13g.

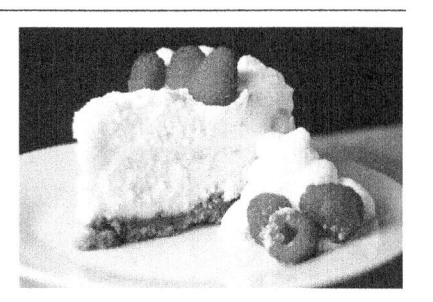

Ingredients:

Cream cheese	16oz.
Egg	2
Vanilla bean, scraped	1 medium
Vanilla extract	1 tsp.
Sugar	½ cup

Cooking procedure:

1. Place all the ingredients in your blender. Blend well. Do not place the whole bean, scrape the seeds out.
2. Now put the blended mixture into a springform pan. Cover it securely with foil. Then, pour two cups of water and place your springform pan on the trivet.
3. Set the time for 20 minutes. Let it cook.
4. Remove from instant pot and cool. Chill in the refrigerator before serving.

Simple Brownie Cake

Overall cooking time: 30 min

Servings: 4

Nutrition info: Calories: 400, fat: 14g, Carbs: 54g, protein: 3g.

Ingredients:

Butter	4 tbsp.
Chocolate chips	2 tbsp.
Sugar	2/3 cup
Egg	2
Vanilla extract	¼ cup
All-purpose flour	½ cup
Cocoa powder	4 tbsp.
Powdered sugar	2 tbsp.

Cooking procedure:

1. Take a microwave safe bowl and place the butter and chocolate chips into it. Transfer it to the microwave for 1 minute to melt the butter.
2. Beat the butter and chocolate chips in a large mixing bowl. Add sugar and beat. Break the eggs into it; add the vanilla extract and beat until smooth. Add the flour, cocoa, and mix well.
3. Now place the rack in your instant pot and cover it with foil. Add the mixture.
4. Close the lid and set the time for 18 minutes at high pressure.
5. Top with powdered sugar and serve.

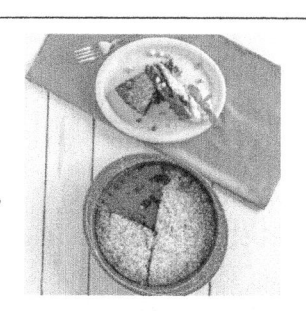

Paleo Chocolate Cake

Overall cooking time: 20 min

Servings: 2-3

Nutrition info: Calories: 250, fat: 16g, Carbs: 20g, protein: 6g.

Ingredients:

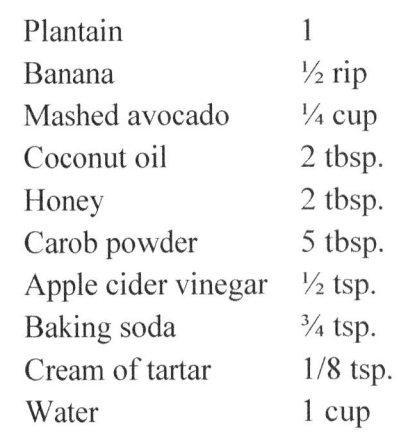

Plantain	1
Banana	½ rip
Mashed avocado	¼ cup
Coconut oil	2 tbsp.
Honey	2 tbsp.
Carob powder	5 tbsp.
Apple cider vinegar	½ tsp.
Baking soda	¾ tsp.
Cream of tartar	1/8 tsp.
Water	1 cup

Cooking procedure:

1. Place the banana, plantain, honey, coconut oil, avocado, cream of tartar, baking soda, vinegar and carob into a blender. Blend until making a smooth mixture.
2. Now, grease three or four ramekins with coconut oil and fill them about ¾ full.
3. In your instant pot, place the steaming rack and pour the water. Then arrange the pans on the rack.
4. Close the lid and set the time for 18 minutes.
5. Make a topping of coconut flakes, coconut cream or fruit.

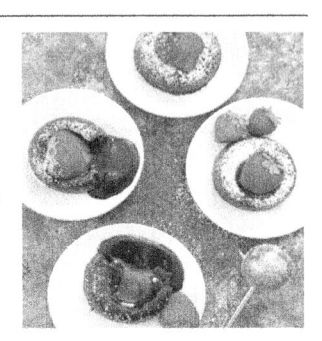

Healthy Apple Crisp

Overall cooking time: 12 min

Servings: 4

Nutrition info: Calories: 200, fat: 14g, Carbs: 13g, protein: 3g.

Ingredients:

Apple	5
Cinnamon	2 tbsp.
Nutmeg	½ tbsp.
Water	½ cup
Maple syrup	1 tbsp.
Butter	4 tbsp.
Old fashioned oats	2/4 cup
Flour	¼ cup
Brown sugar	¼ cup
Salt	½ tsp.

Cooking procedure:

1. Place the apples in your instant pot. Sprinkle the cinnamon and nutmeg over them, then the water and maple syrup.
2. In a microwave safe bowl, melt the butter in your microwave and then transfer it to a mixing bowl. Add the oats, brown sugar, salt, and flour. Mix evenly. Now drop the mixture into the top of the apples.
3. Close the lid and manually set the time for 8 minutes at high pressure.
4. Release the pressure and leave it to sit a little.
5. Serve hot with a topping of vanilla ice cream.

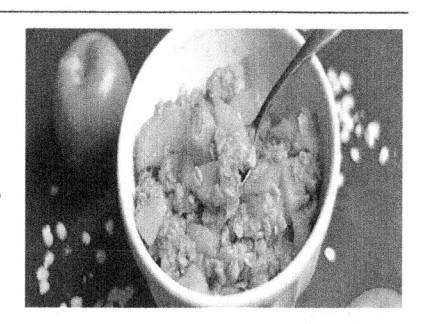

Mouthwatering Orange Cheesecake

Overall cooking time: 30 min

Servings: 8

Nutrition info: Calories: 375, fat: 24g, Carbs: 32g, protein: 3.7g.

Ingredients:

For the nut crust
Blanched almond flour	1 ½ cups
Sweetener	1 ½ tbsp.
Butter	3 tbsp.

For orange cheesecake filling:

Packaged cream cheese	8oz.
Pastured eggs	2
Sweetener	½ cup
Vanilla extract	tbsp.
Orange juice	4 tbsp.
Orange zest	2 tbsp.

Cooking procedure:

1. Preheat your oven to 350-degrees F. In a mixing bowl, mix the nut crust ingredients and then place into stackable pans.
2. Bake for 10 minutes. Remove from oven.
3. To make the cheesecake filling, add all ingredients of the filling into a blender and blend well.
4. Place the trivet in your instant pot and then pour in 2 cups of water. Cover the trivet to prevent evaporation.
5. Now, pour the filling mixture into springform pans. Place the pans onto the trivet. Cover with aluminum foil.

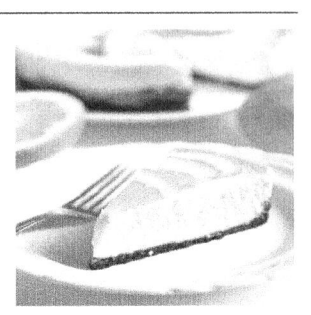

6. Close the lid and set the time for 25 minutes at high pressure.
7. Chill thoroughly. Top with above and serve.

Pina Colada Rice Pudding

Overall cooking time: 15 min

Servings: 8

Nutrition info: Calories: 160, fat: 0g, Carbs: 27g, protein: 10g.

Ingredients:

White rice	1 cup
Water	1 ½ cup
Coconut oil	1 tbsp.
Salt	¼ tsp.
Coconut milk	14oz
Sugar	½ cup
Eggs	2
Half-and-half	½ cup
Vanilla extract	1 tsp.

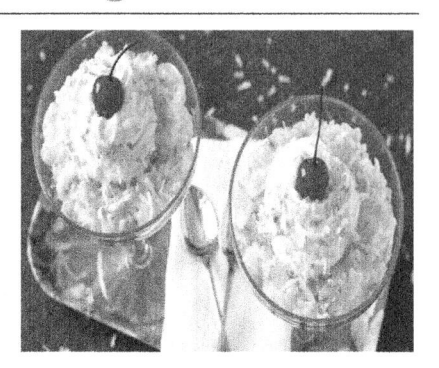

Cooking procedure:

1. Place the rice, coconut oil, and the water in the instant pot and combine. Set the time for 5 minutes at high pressure.
2. When it is done, open the lid and add the sugar and milk into the pot.
3. In a mixing bowl, break the eggs add the half-and-half and the vanilla extract and mix well. Pour slowly the mixture into the pot and stir continuously.
4. Now turn on the sauté button of your instant pot and continue stirring to thicken.
5. Pour onto a serving plate.

Delicious Pumpkin Pies

Overall cooking time: 15 min

Servings: 8

Nutrition info: Calories: 143, fat: 2.4g, Carbs: 29g, protein: 3.3g.

Ingredients:

Butternut squash	2 lbs.
Whole milk	1 cup
Maple syrup	¾ cup
Eggs	2
Powdered cinnamon	1 tbsp.
Powdered ginger	½ tsp.
Powdered cloves	¼ tsp.
Corn starch	1 tbsp.
Sea salt	2 pinches

Cooking procedure:

1. First, prepare your instant pot and add one cup of water and the squash cubes.
2. Close the lid and set the time for 4 minutes at high pressure.
3. Meanwhile, in a mixing bowl, add the maple syrup, milk, ginger, salt, cornstarch, cinnamon, eggs and beat them all together.
4. When the cooking is done, open up the lid and mash the squash through a fine mesh strainer.
5. Measure the pumpkin pulp by putting it into a cup, combine the pumpkin with the egg mixture, and mix.

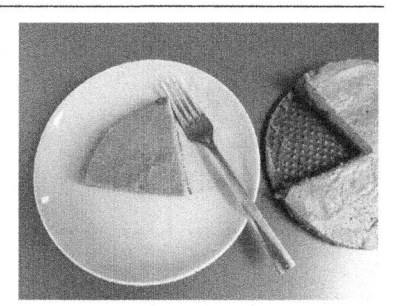

Easy Oreo Cheesecake

Overall cooking time: 55 min

Servings: 6

Nutrition info: Calories: 150, fat: 9.5g, Carbs: 15g, protein: 2g.

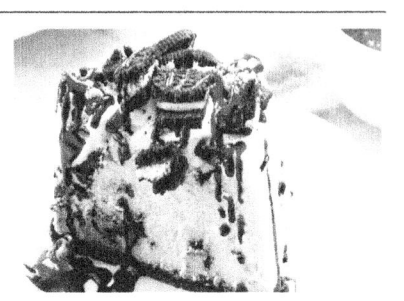

Ingredients:

For the crust
Whole Oreo cookies	12
Salted butter	2 tbsp.

For the cheesecake

Cream cheese	16 oz.
Granulated sugar	½ cup
Eggs	2
All-purpose flour	1 tbsp.
Heavy cream	¼ cup
Pure vanilla extract	2 tbsp.
Oreo cookies	8

Cooking procedure:

1. Take the springform pan first, wrap tightly in foil, and spray with a non-stick cooking spray.
2. In a mixing bowl, add the Oreo cookies with melted butter and place it into the pan. Freeze for 10 minutes.
3. Now, take a large bowl and beat the cream cheese evenly. Add the sugar, eggs, flour, vanilla extract and then the heavy cream. Make sure that you do it successively. Fold the crushed Oreo cookies in.

4. Place the butter into the pan and cover the pan with aluminum foil. Pour ½ cup water and place the trivet.
5. Here, arrange the cheesecake into the pan and close the lid. Manually set the time of the instant pot to 40 minutes at high pressure.
6. Separate the cake from the instant pot gently and remove the foil from the cheesecake.
7. Cool and top before serving.

Delicious Tapioca Pudding

Overall cooking time: 20 min

Servings: 4-6

Nutrition info: Calories: 187, fat: 2.5g, Carbs: 29g, protein: 2.5g.

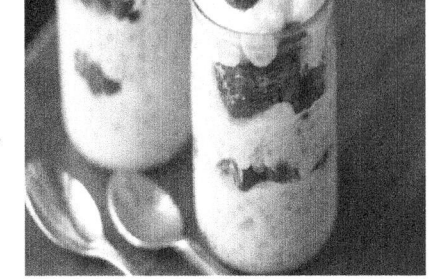

Ingredients:

Seed tapioca	½ cup
Whole milk	1 ¼ cups
Water	½ cup
Sugar	½ cup
Lemon zest	½ cup

Cooking procedure:

1. First, prepare your instant pot by adding a cup of water into it and placing the trivet.
2. Now in a heatproof bowl, add the tapioca seeds and the milk, lemon zest, sugar, and water. Combine well.
3. Place the bowl on the trivet in the instant pot and close the lid. Set the time for 8 minutes at high pressure.
4. When the cooking is done, lift out your item and spoon into several serving cups.

Easy Banana Bread

Overall cooking time: 55 min

Servings: 4

Nutrition info: Calories: 155, fat: 6g, Carbs: 24g, protein: 3g.

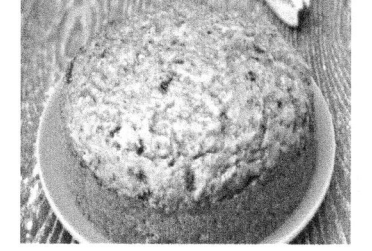

Ingredients:

Mashed banana	4
Soft butter	1 slice
Vanilla	1 tbsp.
Egg	2
Sugar	½ cup
Flour	2 cups
Baking powder	1 tbsp.

Cooking procedure:

1. Take a mixing bowl and break the eggs into it. Add the butter and sugar and mix thoroughly. Now add the mashed banana and vanilla. Stir.
2. Combine the butter and flour in a separate mixing bowl and then add the dry ingredients to the wet and combine well.
3. Now pour the mixture into few springform pans and place them on the trivet of an instant pot where a cup of water has already been added.

Soup Recipes

Butternut Squash Soup

Overall cooking time: 20 min

Servings: 6

Nutrition info: Calories: 90, fat: 2g, Carbs: 17g, protein: 2g.

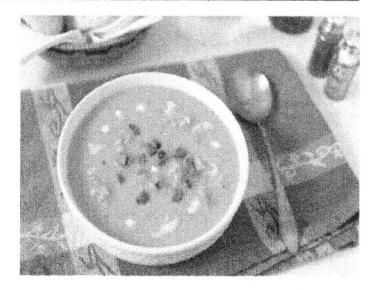

Ingredients:

Olive oil	1 tbsp.
Yellow onion	1 large
Bell pepper	1
Garlic	2 tbsp.
Ground ginger	1 tsp.
Butternut squash	2 lbs.
Apple	1 medium

Sage	1 tbsp.
Chili powder	1/8 tsp.
Sea salt	¼ tsp.
Chicken stock	3 cup
Goat cheese	3 oz.
Parmesan cheese	½ cup
Salted pepitas	for topping

Cooking procedure:

1. Set the sauté function on your instant pot and add the olive oil. Add the onion and bell pepper and sauté for 4 minutes. Add the ginger and garlic and stir for 1 minute more using the sauté function.
2. Now add the chicken stock, chili powder, sage, apple, cubed squash and sea salt into the instant pot and close the lid. Set the time for 5 minutes at high pressure.
3. After cooking, puree everything with an immersion blender. Add the cheese and mix to make it smooth.
4. Serve with some pepitas on top.

Curried Butternut Squash Soup

Overall cooking time: 20 min

Servings: 6

Nutrition info: Calories: 90, fat: 1g, Carbs: 18g, protein: 3g.

Ingredients:

Butternut squash	1
Onion	1, chopped
Garlic	2 cloves
Ginger	1 tbsp.
Curry powder	2 tsp.
Olive oil	2 tbsp.
Coconut milk	14oz.
Vegetable stock	4 cups
Salt and pepper	to taste

Cooking procedure:

1. Press the sauté function of your instant pot and add the olive oil. A minute later, add the onion and sauté until softened, then add the ginger, garlic, curry powder, pepper, and salt. Sauté and stir.
2. Now add the butternut squash cubes and sauté for 2 to 3 minutes. Pour in the vegetable stock and coconut milk. Close the lid and set the time for 12 minutes at high pressure.
3. When it is done, blend the soup to make it creamy using an immersion blender.

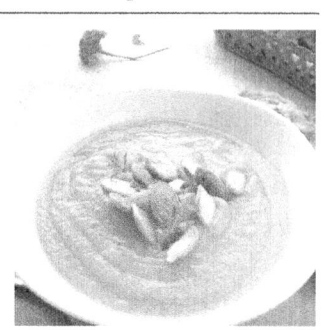

Healthy Keto Chili

Overall cooking time: 30 min

Servings: 8-10

Nutrition info: Calories: 306, fat: 18g, Carbs: 14g, protein: 23g.

Ingredients:

Beef	2 lbs.
Onion	1, chopped
Garlic	8 cloves
Tomatoes	8-10, chopped
Chilies	4 oz.
Worcestershire sauce	2 tbsp.
Chili powder	¼ cup
Cumin	2 tbsp.
Oregano	1 tbsp.
Sea salt	2 tbsp.
Black pepper	1 tbsp.
Bay leaf	1

Cooking procedure:

1. Turn on the sauté function of your instant pot. Add the oil and the onion and sauté to make the onion translucent. Add the garlic and cook for 1 minute more.
2. Add the ground beef and sauté for 8 to 10 minutes. Add the remaining ingredients.
3. Close the lid and press the cancel button on your instant pot. Press the Meat button for pressure cooking for 30 minutes.
4. Release the pressure and then open the lid and place the item on a serving plate.

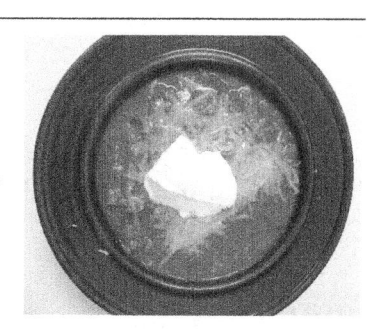

Bean and Sausage Soup

Overall cooking time: 55 min

Servings: 8-10

Nutrition info: Calories: 390, fat: 14g, Carbs: 34g, protein: 27g.

Ingredients:

Black-eyed peas	2 cups
Chicken stock	4 cups
Chicken sausage	12 oz.
Leek	1, chopped
Rosemary	1 large
Garlic	3 cloves
Tomatoes	15 oz., crushed.
Worcestershire sauce	2 tbsp.
Bay leaves	2

Cooking procedure:

1. Take your instant pot and place the black-eyed peas and the chicken stock into it.
2. Close the lid and manually set the time for 25 minutes.
3. When cooking is done, release the pressure and add all remaining ingredients. Again, close the lid and press the soup button for 30 minutes.
4. Release the pressure quickly and serve with your love.

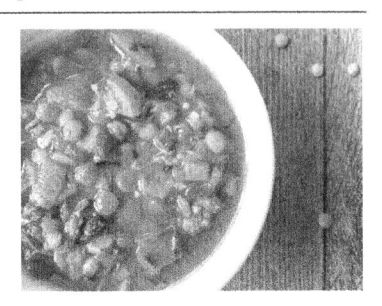

Taco Beef Soup

Overall cooking time: 30 min

Servings: 6

Nutrition info: Calories: 403, fat: 18g, Carbs: 12g, protein: 46g.

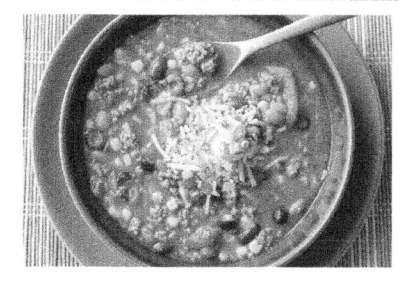

Ingredients:

Coconut oil	1 ½ tbsp.
Yellow onion	1
Bell pepper	4
Ground beef	2 lbs.
Chili powder	2-3 tbsp.
Spices you want	4-6 tbsp.
Sea salt and pepper	to taste.
Tomatoes	8, chopped
Bone broth	24 oz.
Coconut milk	5 oz.

Cooking procedure:

1. Turn on the sauté function of your instant pot. Add the oil, the onion and bell pepper and sauté until the onion is translucent.
2. Add the beef and sauté to make it brown. Pour into a colander and place back into the pot.
3. Add the spice ingredients and stir well, also add the tomatoes, green chilies, broth and coconut milk.
4. Close the lid and manually set the time to 25 minutes after pressing the button Soup.
5. Top as you like and serve.

Homemade Seafood Gumbo

Overall cooking time: 20 min

Servings: 8

Nutrition info: Calories: 346, fat:12g, Carbs: 9g, protein: 49g.

Ingredients:

Sea bass filets	24 oz.
Avocado oil	3 tbsp.
Cajun seasoning	3 tbsp.
Onion	2
Bell peppers	2
Celery ribs	4
Tomatoes	26oz, diced
Tomato paste	¼ cup
Bay leaves	3
Bone broth	1 ½ cups
Shrimp	2 lbs.
Salt and pepper	to taste

Cooking procedure:

1. First, season the sea bass with Cajun seasoning, salt and pepper. Mix well.
2. Turn on the sauté function of your instant pot and pour in the oil. Add the sea bass chunks and sauté for 4 minutes. Set aside.
3. Now add onion, celery and pepper to the instant pot and sauté for 2 minutes. Add the fish, tomato paste, bay leaves, bone broth and diced tomatoes and stir.
4. Close the lid and set the time to 5 minutes manually.

Quick Broccoli Soup

Overall cooking time: 30 min

Servings: 8

Nutrition info: Calories: 117, fat:7g, Carbs: 11g, protein: 3g.

Ingredients:

Broccoli	4 cups
Vegetable broth	8 cups
Russet potato	1, chopped
Leek	1 chopped
Garlic	6 cloves
Salt	1 tbsp.
Black pepper	½ tsp.

Cooking procedure:

1. Place all the ingredients in the instant pot.
2. Close the lid and manually set the time to 5 minutes at high pressure.
3. After cooking, allow the soup to cool and, using an immersion blender, blend the soup to make it creamy.
4. You are ready to serve.

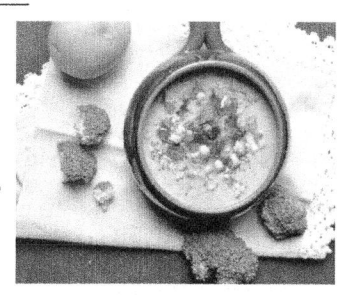

Easy Chicken Soup

Overall cooking time: 45 min

Servings: 6

Nutrition info: Calories: 455, fat: 32g, Carbs: 12g, protein: 29g.

Ingredients:

Chicken thighs	6
Avocado oil	2 tbsp.
Onion	1 medium
Carrots	3, chopped
Celery ribs	3, chopped
Chicken broth	4 cups
Bay leaves	2
Pepper & salt	to taste
Parsley	1, dried
Garlic	2 cloves
Thyme	1, dried

Cooking procedure:

1. Turn on the sauté function of your instant pot and add the olive oil. When heated, add the chicken thighs and brown it on both side. Set aside.
2. Add one teaspoon oil to the instant pot and sauté the carrots, onion and celery ribs for another 2 minutes.
3. Now, add the vegetables and then pour the broth into a cup of water. Add the other ingredients in the instant pot and set the instant pot to Soup mode.
4. When the cooking is done, debone and shred the thighs.

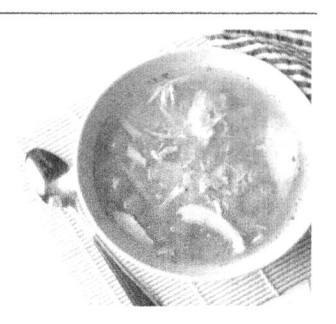

Healthy Carrot Soup

Overall cooking time: 30 min

Servings: 4

Nutrition info: Calories: 133, fat: 5g, Carbs: 20g, protein: 3g.

Ingredients:

Olive oil	1 tbsp.
Onion	1, chopped
Celery	4, chopped
Carrots	2 lbs., sliced
Thyme	handful
Water	4 cups
Chicken	1
Orange juice	½ cup
Lemon juice	1 tbsp.

Salt and pepper to taste.

Cooking procedure:

1. Turn on the sauté function of your instant pot and add the oil. Wait for the oil to heat and then add the onion and sauté until translucent. Then add the garlic and celery. Sauté for 2 minutes. Add carrots and sauté for another 2 minutes.
2. Now add the thyme, bouillon, and water. Close the lid and manually set the time to 10 minutes.
3. Release the pressure and discard the thyme.
4. At the last step, add the orange and lemon juice and blend well.

Tomato Soup

Overall cooking time: 25 min

Servings: 6

Nutrition info: Calories: 154, fat:7g, Carbs: 21g, protein: 5g.

Ingredients:

Butter	3 tbsp.
Onion	2, chopped
Garlic	4 cloves
Carrot	2, coarsely chopped
Tomato paste	2 tbsp.
Bone broth	1 quart
Tomato	5 large
Basil	½ cup
Honey	2 tbsp.
Salt and pepper to taste	

Cooking procedure:

1. Plug in your instant pot and press the sauté function. Add the carrot, onion, salt, and pepper and sauté for 6 to 7 minutes.
2. Then add the tomato paste with garlic. Continue cook for 1 minute more.
3. Now add the tomato, basil, and the bone broth and set the time to 10 minutes after pressing the SOUP button.
4. When the cooking is done, add the honey and blend well.
5. Your soup is ready.

Kale Soup with Chicken and Sweet Potato

Overall cooking time: 20 min

Servings: 6-8

Nutrition info: Calories: 120, fat: 2.4g, Carbs: 13g, protein: 10g.

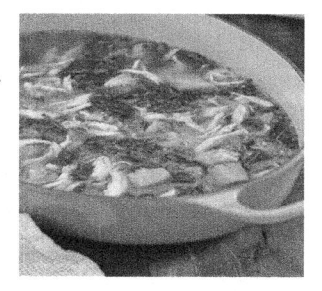

Ingredients:

Sweet potato	3
Chicken broth	90 oz.
Chicken breast	1 pack
Jeo's Mirapoix	1 container
Olive oil	2 tbsp.
Salt and pepper	to taste
Bay kale	one bag
Thyme	to taste

Cooking procedure:

1. Set the sauté function on your instant pot and add the olive oil and the mirapoix. Then add the chicken breasts and cook to brown.
2. Now, add the all other ingredients except the kale. Close the lid and set the time for 8 minutes at high pressure.
3. Release the pressure and add the kale. Cook for 1 minute more at high pressure.
4. Serve.

Homemade Beef Paleo Stew

Overall cooking time: 25 min

Servings: 6

Nutrition info: Calories: 386, fat: 18g, Carbs: 24g, protein: 32g.

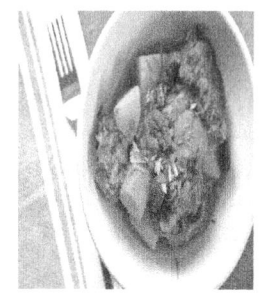

Ingredients:

Stewing beef	2lbs.
Avocado oil	2 tbsp.
Crimini mushrooms	3 cups
Russet potatoes	3
Parsnip	2 cups
Celery	3 stalks
Tapioca flour	2 tbsp.
Beef stock	1 liter
Sherry vinegar	3 tbsp.
Parsley	4 stalks
Carrots	3, chopped
Salt and pepper	to taste

Cooking procedure:

1. Go to the sauté function on your instant pot and add the oil. Add the beef with salt and pepper. Brown the meat. Set aside.
2. Add a little oil to the instant pot and add the mushrooms, carrots, celery, and shallot and sauté for 2 minutes. Add the tomato and sauté for another minute.
3. Now add the potatoes and the parsnip. Also, add the beef and juices.
4. In a mixing bowl, mix the tapioca flour with ¼ cup hot water and add it to the instant pot. Add the beef stockand other ingredients if you want.
5. Set the cover and cook for 30 minutes at high pressure.

Apple Soup with Butternut Squash

Overall cooking time: 25 min

Servings: 6

Nutrition info: Calories: 180, fat: 11g, Carbs: 19g, protein: 2g.

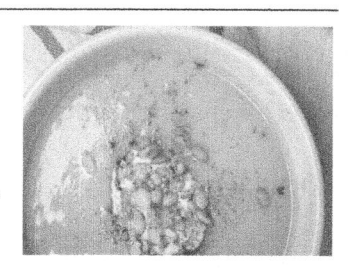

Ingredients:

Butternut squash	1, cubed
Apple	1
Ginger powder	2 tbsp.
Chicken broth	4 cups
Olive oil	to taste

Cooking procedure:

1. Go to sauté button on your instant pot. Add the oil and butternut squash and brown it evenly.
2. Now add the other ingredients. Close the lid and set the time to 10 minutes at high pressure.
3. Use an immersion blender to puree the soup.

Broccoli and Cheddar Soup

Overall cooking time: 25 min

Servings: 6

Nutrition info: Calories: 117, fat: 7g, Carbs: 11g, protein: 3g.

Ingredients:

Fresh broccoli	2 heads, chopped
Chicken broth	4 cups
Heavy cream	1 cup
Cheddar cheese	2 cups
Salt and pepper	to taste.

Cooking procedure:

1. Take your instant pot and add the broccoli and broth. Close the lid and manually set the time for 3 minutes at high pressure.
2. When cooking is done quickly release the pressure, open the lid and add the other ingredients.
3. Puree the soup until smooth.

Easy Chicken Noodle Soup with

Spinach

Overall cooking time: 40 min

Servings: 6

Nutrition info: Calories: 227, fat: 6g, Carbs: 19g, protein: 22g.

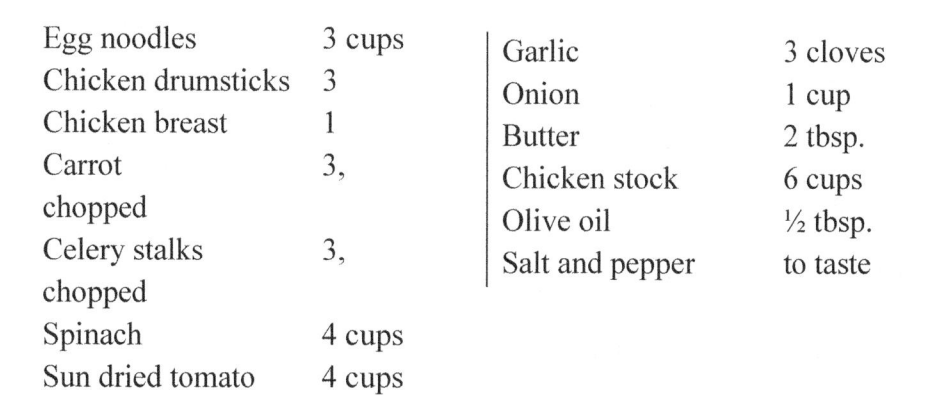

Ingredients:

Egg noodles	3 cups	Garlic	3 cloves
Chicken drumsticks	3	Onion	1 cup
Chicken breast	1	Butter	2 tbsp.
Carrot chopped	3,	Chicken stock	6 cups
Celery stalks chopped	3,	Olive oil	½ tbsp.
Spinach	4 cups	Salt and pepper	to taste
Sun dried tomato	4 cups		

Cooking procedure:

1. Turn on the sauté function and add the olive oil. Add the garlic and onion and sauté for 2 minutes.
2. Now add the carrots, spinach, and celery and cook until soft. Then add the butter, chicken and the stock to the pot.
3. Close the lid and manually set the cook time for 10 minutes.
4. Remove the chicken from the instant pot and turn the instant pot back to the sauté function. Add the tomatoes and the egg noodles. Cook until the noodles soften. Shred the chicken and add the noodles. Add salt and pepper.

Easy Beef and Leek Soup

Overall cooking time: 25 min

Servings: 4

Nutrition info: Calories: 98, fat: 4g, Carbs: 14g, protein: 1.3g.

Ingredients:

Olive oil	2 tbsp.
Shallots	2, chopped
Garlic	2 cloves
Ginger	1 tbsp.
Leek	1, sliced
Beets	1 ½ lbs.
Turmeric	1 tbsp.
Paprika	1 tsp.
Coconut milk	1 can
Salt and pepper to taste	

Cooking procedure:

1. Tenderize the shallots with garlic and ginger for 5 minutes using the sauté function pf your instant pot. Then add the beets, paprika, salt, and pepper and mix well.
2. Now add the vegetable stock and the milk and stir.
3. Close the lid and turn on the SOUP function. Adjust the time to 15 minutes.
4. Blend the soup when it is cool enough for you to enjoy it.

Breakfast Recipes

Healthy Coconut Yogurt

Overall cooking time: 15 hours and 5 min

Servings: 6

Nutrition info: Calories: 170, fat: 1.4g, Carbs: 33g, protein: 5g.

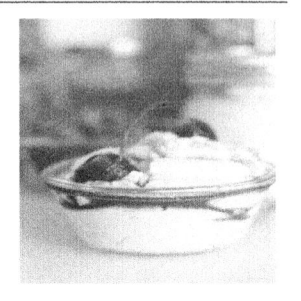

Ingredients:

Coconut cream   2 cans
Probiotic   4 capsules

Cooking procedure:

1. First, pour the coconut cream into the cooker. Press the Yogurt button and when it comes to a boil, open the lid and watch the temperature. When the temperature reaches 120 F, open the capsules and add the powder to the instant pot. Stir to mix the powder with the cream.
2. Close the lid and press the yogurt button. Adjust the time to 15 hours. Leave.
3. When finished, pour the yogurt into a bowl and transfer to your refrigerator for a day.

Oatmeal with Caramelized Bananas

Overall cooking time: 20 min

Servings: 4

Nutrition info: Calories: 330, fat: 12g, Carbs: 51g, protein: 7g.

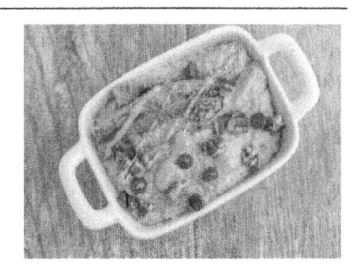

Ingredients:

Oats	1 cup
Milk	1 cup
Water	1.5 cups
Peanut butter	1/3 cup
Bananas	2
Butter	1 tbsp.

Cooking procedure:

1. Put the first three ingredients into the instant pot and close the lid. Manually set the time for 8 minutes at high pressure. Allow to cook.
2. Meanwhile, slice the banana and melt the butter.
3. Turn off the cooker and naturally release the pressure. Add the butter and stir well.
4. Serve with topping of banana and chocolate chips.

Easy Homemade Oats

Overall cooking time: 12 min

Servings: 4

Nutrition info: Calories: 140, fat: 2.5g, Carbs: 26g, protein: 4g.

Ingredients:

Steel cut oats	1 cup
Brown sugar	¼ cup
Butter	2 tbsp.
Salt	1 pinch
Water	3 cups
Cranberries	½ cup
Slivered almonds	½ cup

Cooking procedure:

1. Take your instant pot and add the butter, brown sugar, salt, water, and oats. Stir and close the lid. Set the cooking time to 12 minutes.
2. Release the pressure and stir to desired consistency.
3. Serve with topping of cranberries and almonds.

Healthy Instant Oats with Fruit

Overall cooking time: 15 min

Servings: 2

Nutrition info: Calories: 98, fat: 4g, Carbs: 14g, protein: 1.3g.

Ingredients:

Steel cut oats	1 cup
Water	1. 5 cups.
Butter	2 tbsp.
Orange juice	1 cup
Cranberries	1 tbsp.
Raisins	1 tbsp.
Dried apricots	1 tbsp.
Maple syrup	2 tbsp.
Cinnamon	¼ tsp.
Pecans	2 tbsp.
Salt	to taste

Cooking procedure:

1. Add the all ingredients in the instant pot and stir to combine well. Close the lid and manually set the time for 10 minutes.
2. Open the cover, stir everything and transfer to the serving cups.

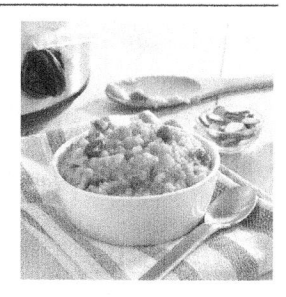

Energetic Boiled Egg

Overall cooking time: 15 min

Servings: 2

Nutrition info: Calories: 60, fat: 4g, Carbs: 0g, protein: 6g.

Ingredients:

Egg   2
Water   1 cup

Cooking procedure:

1. Take your instant pot and add the rack comes with it. Pour in 1 cup of water and then add the eggs.
2. Close the lid and set the time for 10 minutes at high pressure.
3. Release the pressure as you want and then separate the egg from the water to cool. Peel and cut in half.

Banana French Toast

Overall cooking time: 20 min

Servings: 4

Nutrition info: Calories: 180, Fat: 5g, Carbs: 31g, Protein: 5g.

Ingredients:

Butter	1 tbsp.
Steel cut oats	1 cup
Water	3 cups
Salt	to taste
Raisins	¾ cup

Cooking procedure:

1. Turn on to sauté function and add the butter. When it is melted, add the toast and the oats. Stir and make it dark.
2. Now add the water and salt. Stir and close the lid. Manually set the time for 10 minutes.
3. When it is done, remove the lid and stir with raisins. Sit for 5 to 10 minutes to allow the oats thicken.
4. Serve with your favorite topping.

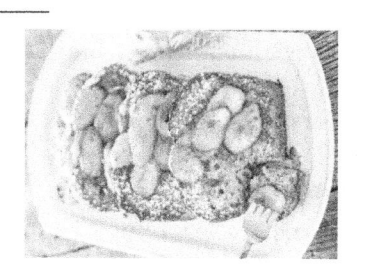

Delicious Scotch Eggs

Overall cooking time: 30 min

Servings: 4

Nutrition info: Calories: 288, fat: 16g, Carbs: 1g, protein: 27g.

Ingredients:

Egg	4
Ground sausage	1lb.
Vegetable oil	1 tbsp.

Cooking procedure:

1. Take your instant pot and add the rack that came with it. Pour in 1 cup of water and then place the eggs.
2. Close the lid and set the time for 10 minutes at high pressure.
3. Release the pressure as you want and then separate the eggs from the water to cool. Peel and wrap the eggs with the sausages around the eggs.
4. Remove the rack and set the instant pot to sauté function and sauté the eggs in the vegetable oil. Set aside.
5. Set the rack back in the instant pot and add the water. Now place the eggs and set the time for 6 minutes.
6. Yap, ready.

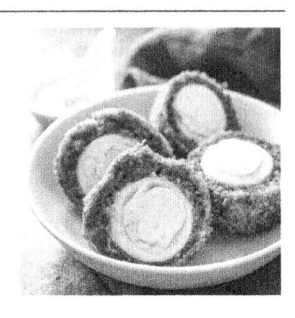

Delicious Yogurt with Fruit

Overall cooking time: 8 hours and 30 min

Servings: 6

Nutrition info: Calories: 232, fat: 0.5g, Carbs: 34g, protein: 10g.

Ingredients:

Milk	1 gallon
Greek yogurt	½ cup
Vanilla bean paste	2 tbsp.
Fruit	2 cups
Sugar	1 cup

Cooking procedure:

1. Pour the milk into your instant pot and press the yogurt button. Set the time for 45 minutes.
2. Turn off the cooker and when it reaches 115 F, add the yogurt and the vanilla bean paste.
3. Turn on the instant pot and set the yogurt button again. Allow to cook for 8 hours.
4. Transfer the yogurt into convenient sized jar and place in the refrigerator. Leave it for 1-day.
5. When you are about to serve, boil the fruit with the sugar and cool before serving.
6. Place the yogurt in the serving cup and place the fruit on the top of the yogurt.

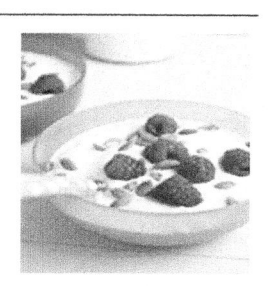

Breakfast Quinoa

Overall cooking time: 30 min

Servings: 6

Nutrition info: Calories: 400, fat: 2g, Carbs: 22g, protein: 7g.

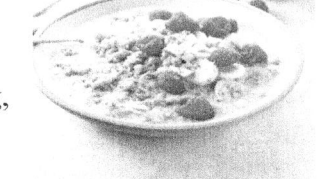

Ingredients:

Quinoa	1 ½ cups
Water	2 ¼ cups
Maple syrup	2 tbsp.
Vanilla	½ tbsp.
Cinnamon	¼ tsp.
Salt	to taste

Cooking procedure:

1. Add all the ingredients into the instant pot and close the lid. Manually set the time to 1 minute at high pressure. Allow to cook.
2. Turn off the cooker and naturally release the pressure.
3. Fluff and serve with berries, milk and sliced almonds.

Easy Buckwheat Porridge

Overall cooking time: 30 min

Servings: 4

Nutrition info: Calories: 300, Fat: 14g, Carbs: 34g, Protein: 7g.

Ingredients:

Raw buckwheat groats	1 cup
Rice milk	3 cups
Banana	1, sliced
Raisins	¼ cup
Ground cinnamon	1 tsp.
Vanilla	½ tsp.

Cooking procedure:

1. Place the buckwheat, cinnamon, vanilla, raisins, banana and rice milk into the instant pot.
2. Secure the lid and set the time for 6 minutes at high pressure.
3. When the cooking is done, allow naturally release the pressure and then stir the porridge.
4. When it is time to serve, add more rice milk to get the desire consistency.

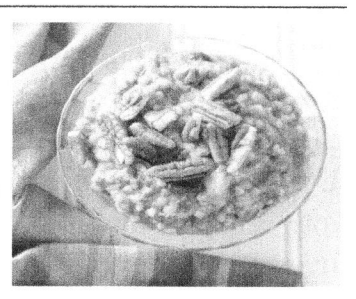

CONCLUSION

To conclude, I want to tell you the main reason why you should choose the instant pot as a crucial utensil in your kitchen and the health benefits of everything you can cook in it. The real question is, why we should we choose the Instant Pot? With a minimal investment in this product, the return on investment is astronomical. Not only are you saving money by not buying other cooking products because the Instant Pot is such an inclusive cooker, but you are saving time and energy during your busy day as well.

With the numerous features provided, we have not seen a dish that cannot be prepared by the Instant Pot. So, decide what cravings you want to cure, gather the ingredients, choose your recipe, sit back and relax, then enjoy your delicious meal. Thank you for reading my cookbook, and I hope you will use all the acquired knowledge productively.

Made in the USA
Monee, IL
07 December 2020